RESET

You are in: **CONTROL**

Change your perspective: **ALT**

Forget the past: **DELETE**

BRIAN MICHAEL GOOD

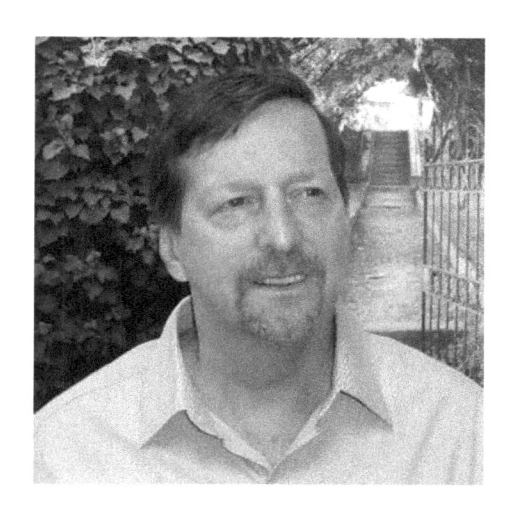

BRIAN MICHAEL GOOD

Author – Writer – Entrepreneur

A Genius, Autistic, Empath, and Savant

"I believe it is more important to write quality books, not a quantity of books. I put part of my heart and soul into the writing of 'Never Surrender Your Soul', 'RESET: Control, Alt, Delete', and 'Quotes Of Wisdom To Live By', as an artist puts part of their heart and soul into their work of art."

– Brian Michael Good

I have lived a life buffeted by character-altering hurricanes. My life storms began in my trauma-filled childhood within my dysfunctional family.

My childhood was filled with tension, excessive discipline, and yelling – at home and at grammar school – each contributed to a lower self-esteem and academic performance during my formative developmental years. Yelling and corporal punishment instilled fear in me. I carried such sentiments and emotional trauma with me into adulthood.

I accepted the abuse that I allowed others to bestow on me. It took me a lifetime to discover that I was a Genius, Autistic, Empath, and Savant.

I survived a childhood of verbal, physical, and sexual abuse; dealt with depression, PTSD, the death of two siblings. A bit further on in life, there was the stigma of being homeless not once, but three times, and bankruptcy two times. I was also diagnosed with a six-pound cancerous tumor that was doubling in size every two months. A suicide attempt in 2003 nearly cost me my life. The death of my best friend, three divorces, and the rejection of my only daughter was to follow.

Psychics and people of faith say that we all come back, and some of us come back to teach a lesson. The homeless person on the street has sacrificed their life to teach compassion and tolerance to others. The homeless person, if he or she would know this, might ask, why should I try to improve my life if I came back to suffer to teach this lesson?

The answer is that if one is spiritual, the suffering is only part of the lesson. The most important part is to overcome. We must examine our flaws and try to fix them. Then, in the next chapter of our life, we come back to a better existence.

How can one man encounter so many hurricanes, survive them, learn from them, and then strive to make the world around him a better place? This was the question Brian asked himself that led to this book. I have a deep sense of compassion and empathy for others; social virtues that I value most in my life.

What I have learned from my personal experience can give you hope. You are not alone and you are not forgotten. Your life will improve. Peace and happiness are renewed for those who seek it. I believe that you too will find wisdom in the pearls that have washed ashore as a result of my hurricanes and count yourself a survivor.

Author of "Never Surrender Your Soul – your very essence," "RESET: Control, Alt, Delete," and "Quotes of Wisdom to Live By".

Founder of *Nutricare Plus*, *Tattoo You Aftercare*, and the *Best to Live Foundation* is a 501(c) (3) not-for-profit organization.

Nutricare Plus and *Tattoo You AfterCare* markets natural health and healing by offering special formulated skin care products, herbal remedies for the body, mind, and spirit using only the highest quality of herbal, natural, and organic ingredients.

The *Best To Live Foundation* is a 501(c)(3) not-for-profit organization whose goal is to be an outreach initiative providing answers, information, and provide resources for health needs and overall wellness for anyone who needs to survive emotional, mental, or physical stress.

Credits

Art/Design: Book Front Cover and Back by Daniela Owergoor

www.SelfPubBookCovers.com/Daniela

10% of the "Never Surrender Your Soul" and "RESET: Control, Alt, Delete" book's profits will be donated to *The Best To Live Foundation*, a 501(c)(3) not-for-profit if an equal amount is match by the donations of others.

www.BestToLive.org/Donate.html

*Take the "**Best To Live Lemon-Aid Challenge**"*
to Help Stop Self-Harm

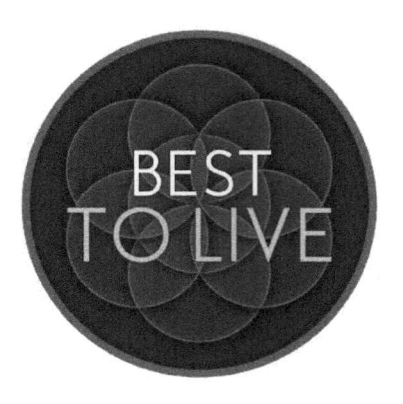

We need to talk about lemons, in other words, Help Stop Self-Harm. We would like you to take the #B2LLemonAidCHL, as a way to raise money for the *Best to Live* Non-Profit. We challenge you to eat three slices of lemon or donate $10.00 to *Best to Live*. It is our hope that by supporting self-harmers they might eat three slices of lemon and forget why they were about to cut themselves.

Copyright © 2014 by Brian Michael Good
First Edition – published 7/24/2015
ISBN: 978-0-9862527-6-1

All rights renewed. No part of this publication may be reproduced, distributed, or transmitted in any form or by any means, including, but not limited to: photocopying, recording, or other electronic or mechanical methods, without the prior written permission of the publisher, except in the case of brief quotations embodied in critical reviews and certain other noncommercial uses permitted by copyright law. For permission requests, write to the Big Bang Publishing, "Attention: Permissions Coordinator," at the following address.

Big Bang Publishing
Attention: Permissions Coordinator
3311 Gulf Breeze Parkway, # 133
Gulf Breeze, Florida 32563

BIG BANG

PUBLISHING

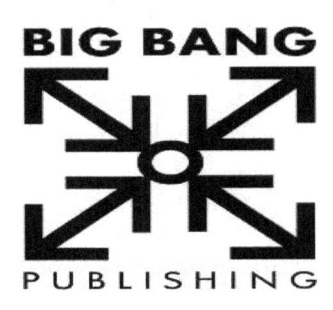

"RESET: Control, Alt, Delete" can be purchased for educational, business, sales promotions, youth groups, personal growth, self-help, positive thinking, happiness, motivational, success, inspirational, finding your destiny, self-fulfillment use, mental illness, depression, anxiety, or fear. Inquire about a wholesale price from a distributor or Big Bang Publisher at the address above.

Disclaimer

Content and information contained in "Reset, Control, Alt, Delete" is not a substitute for professional medical advice, counseling, diagnosis, or treatment. Nor is it intended to replace a consultation with a qualified medical professional. Never delay or disregard seeking professional medical or mental health advice from your physician or other qualified health provider because of something you have read about in "Reset, Control, Alt, Delete." Brian Michael Good, "Author" and Big Bang Publishing do not diagnose, prescribe or treat anyone medically.

"Reset, Control, Alt, Delete" is designed to provide inspiration to reader's world-wide. It is sold with the understanding that the author and publisher are not engaged to render any type of psychological, legal, financial or any other form of professional advice. The content of each chapter is the sole expression and opinion of the author. No warranties or guarantees are expressed or implied by the author. Neither the publisher nor the individual author shall be liable for any physical, psychological, emotional, financial or commercial damages, including, but not limited to, special, incidental, consequential or other damages. The views and rights of the author and publisher are the same: You are responsible for your own choices, actions, and results.

Table of Contents

Introduction	13
Loss of Innocence	17
Finding Happiness	21
Facts of Life	25
Faith, Hope, Belief, Logic, and Knowledge	27
Acceptance is a Gift	31
Fear, Anxiety, Anger, and Depression	33
Healing Yourself	39
Coping Skills	43
Getting a Tune-Up	47
Change	51
Solving Your Problems	53
Control the Present	55
Living in the Present	59
Rebuilding Your Life	63
Find Someone Who Cares	67
Finding Your Destiny	69
I Wanted to Change the World	73
Pearls of Wisdom: Life and Destiny	75
Testicular Cancer	79
Abuse is No Excuse	81
Death at My Door	83
Save a Life	89
Depression – Homelessness – Shelters	91
Thinking about Death by Suicide	93
Play the Hand Life Dealt You	97
Never Surrender	99
About Brian Michael Good	101
Nutricare Plus, Tattoo You, and Best To Live	107
Social Media Links	111
Social Media Connections	113
Thank You	115
The Boot Camp	117
Book Offer	130

Introduction

"Change your world peacefully or your world will change you. You are either the hammer – writer – supplier – leader – speaker or the nail – reader – consumer – follower – audience. The hammer and the nail were designed to build the world together and to create good, not to destroy. Become the positive hammer and nail of change that you would like to see in the world. You can change the future only by implementing change in the present. Start building a better world today."

– Brian Michael Good

Learn how to rise from the ashes of defeat. Survive. Get self-help, embrace positive thinking, live a happier life, and find your destiny.

A well-written self-help book can help you change your perspective allowing you to infuse new activities into your life. Life's most valuable pearls of wisdom that are nourishment for the body, mind, and soul are often found in books.

If you wish for that inner serenity, personal growth, and fulfillment in life, it is possible! *RESET: Control, Alt, Delete*, unlike other self-help books, is written specifically to help you to find the encouragement, strength, and personal growth that you will need to change your perspective with positive thinking so you can live a hopeful life that creates a path allowing you to find your destiny.

RESET: Control, Alt, Delete is a synopsis of his triumphs over life's challenges, hardships, and obstacles and his struggles with mental health, is meant to encourage struggling individuals make sense of the world and find hope to live a meaningful life.

You will decipher the truth about how to find happiness and meet your destiny. If you haven't developed a passion, concept, or goal for your life and an action plan on the best way to achieve it, you will never know whether you could have made it to a place you once thought was impossible. The author asks you to develop a passion based on what you enjoy most in your life. Write it down and let others know about it. Finding your destiny is not just finding out what makes you happy. You need to take the necessary steps to put your life on the right course to develop your passion. Never put your destiny in the hands of a naysayer, don't listen to them.

As you absorb each chapter you will learn that no one can defeat you; you can only defeat yourself. If you face your challenges, hardships, and obstacles with positive thinking, it takes half the effort to overcome them.

You do not have to give up on the dream and your destiny – to a painful and unsatisfying existence. It was Brian's shaking off of others' mistreatment of him that freed him from his suffering. There is hope and a way out! Help yourself by reading *RESET: Control, Alt, Delete*, you will be encouraged to implement a Health – Fitness – Dieting Program that will change your life for the better.

Becoming unstuck and resetting your life reflects the heart of this motivational book, as the author beseeches the reader to consider areas of life that can weigh them down, such as hardship, fear, and depression, which can seek to drive them to give up.

You too do not have to be held captive by fear, anxiety, or depression. What the author has learned from his personal experiences can give you hope. Your life will improve. Peace is for those who seek it.

It took Brian many years to learn the lessons expressed in *RESET: Control, Alt, Delete*. You will find wisdom in the pearls that have washed ashore – as a result of the author's own hurricanes – and count yourself a survivor. It is his hope that you and others know. You are not Alone or Forgotten.

There's always the possibility of a storm on the horizon. Hurricanes are always part of our struggle for existence. Be ready to deal with life's sudden changes. Living in the present and being a survivor will always be how the author stays in the eye of his hurricanes – safe from the storm around him – challenges, hardships, and obstacles are a part of life. The hurricanes keep coming; I gain strength with each pearl of *Wisdom*.

"When one door closes, another opens; but we often look so long and so regretfully upon the closed door, that we do not see the one which has opened for us."

– Alexander Graham Bell

Loss of Innocence

We are all exposed to the harsh realities of life. There is always going to be someone or a group of people who don't like you. Life is not as perfect as you may have once perceived it to be and you have come to realize that people can be very cruel. Loss of innocence does happen to virtually everyone. It is a normal part of growing up. You have been hurt, broken, and disappointed.

How you were raised and how you are treated can affect your self-image and how you are viewed by your classmates. You are not always in control of what happens to you, but you are in control on how you react to it. If someone kicks over your sand castle that you worked on all day, don't get upset; just build a better one. Show them that very little bothers you. How you view your life will help you to survive. Never put your self-esteem in the hands of an abuser by listening to them. No one can defeat you. You can only defeat yourself. No one can truly save you. You must save yourself.

"Accept everything about yourself – I mean everything. You are you and that is the beginning and the end – no apologies, no regrets."

– Clark Moustakas

Only you as an individual can improve the way you are viewed. It begins with how you view yourself. You are in control of how you are perceived by others by realizing that your self-esteem should not be connected with the acceptance of others. How you view yourself should be far more important than what others think of you. You are much better than you think you are. Accepting yourself the way you are is the secret to happiness and finding peace in your life. You can allow your experiences to destroy you or redefine you. Forget about whom they are; accept who you are, and who you can be. That is a choice

---

"If you are comfortable with yourself, others will be comfortable with you."

– Unknown Author

Body language and non-verbal signals can communicate unintentional or negative things about you even before you start talking. A person with a positive and confident self-image holds his head up high and is self-aware of their surroundings whereas a person with a low self-esteem or a poor self-image looks away from others or looks down with their head bowed which causes drooping shoulders.

Where you look as you walk reflects not only in your self-esteem but also in the self-image you project that affects how you are perceived by others. Think of a happy thought or something that you are good at that allows you to walk in a confident manner with a smile. Look straight ahead as you walk, make eye contact whenever you talk or pass someone in the school hallways. How you make eye contact with someone reveals a lot about you and your self-esteem.

"You're braver than you believe, and stronger than you seem, and smarter than you think."

– A.A. Milne

"It's not who you are that holds you back, it's who you think you're not."

– Unknown Author

"Your thoughts create your experience. Your experience creates your reality. Everything you say is a projection and a creation. The words you use have power. You are always placing an order with every word you speak."

– Jodi Cardoza

"No one can make you feel inferior without your consent."

– Eleanor Roosevelt

"What happens is not as important as how you react to what happens."

– Thaddeus Golas

Finding Happiness

If you ever feel that you cannot go on, that you cannot take the pain and hopelessness anymore, my personal experience and what I have learned from it may give you hope.

With *RESET: Control, Alt, Delete*, I want to reach out to you who are down, sad, hopeless, in pain, and who think life is no longer worth living. I want you to know that you are not alone in your experience. Finding where to get more information and support can be critical because your feelings and questions will not go away quickly. There are so many more happy times ahead of you. With this story, I want to reach out to you. I want you to know that you are not alone in your experience. You are not alone and you are not forgotten. You will not be held captive by fear, anxiety, or depression.

"There are visual stimuli influencing your thoughts as to what happiness should be. A form of mind control. Happiness comes from owning your free will by controlling your thoughts with realistic expectations."

— Brian Michael Good

For many of us, it takes decades to realize that happiness comes from within us. Happiness is how our conscious thoughts react in harmony with the external sources and stimuli in our world. I was raised in a family of eight children where I grew up valuing money. I earned money at nine-years-old with a large paper route, stocked shelves at a 7-Eleven store at thirteen-years-old, and cooked at a restaurant at fourteen-years-old. I realized that money gave me temporary happiness. As I matured to an adult, I began not to value money when my inability to sustain a consistent income became my new, but hopefully not permanent, reality.

"Most folks are about as happy as they make up their minds to be."

– Abraham Lincoln

Valuing money less was an important conscious decision for me when I became chronically unemployed or underemployed, and homeless, like millions of people in today's economy. Except for valuing food and a roof over my head, it was my acceptance of not valuing money and non-essential material goods and services that helped me through hard times. Acceptance of failure is not an excuse to give up on any situation. However, sometimes it is necessary to temporarily accept defeat in order to fight the battle another day with a new plan of action. This gives you hope that victory is still attainable…

I chose to watch my diet attentively. I stopped drinking coffee more than once a day; you really have more control than you think. In January, 2009 I stopped eating fast foods on a regular basis, I've tried to have an organic and all natural diet for the last ten years, which means 50% fruits and vegetables by selecting the colors of the rainbow in the produce I eat. I eat my vegetables raw with the skins left on. Why? Because there are more nutrients in the skin than in the fruit or vegetable and you do not receive the fiber when you juice; just make sure you wash the skin well and get most of the chemicals off; then I cut out the seeds and cut up the fruit or vegetables and put it in a blender and have a smooth, comfortable chill while you are listening to your favorite music. The drink is like the fountain of youth or is it a category 4 hurricane for me. (Rarely do I go out for fast food.)

I attempted suicide in October 2003 because I was depressed. I didn't have a treatment plan and I didn't take my medication for depression. A later chapter, "Getting a Tune-up" seeks to educate anyone taking medication for the first time for mental/physical illness, depression, ADHD, eating disorders, panic attacks, and anxiety to develop a sleep – diet – activity – exercise – plan that fits their lifestyle.

A big part of dealing with depression is realizing that you are in control of your own happiness. How you view your life will help you to survive. Happiness is finding peace in our lives. Peace and happiness are renewed for those who seek it. Forgiveness and acceptance are the key. Forgiveness removes fear. When you forgive, you will have made the decision to move forward. Only you can heal yourself. How you view your life will help you to survive. The first step in forgiving others who have hurt you is acknowledging that it was your free will choice to accept the hurt that others bestowed on you. Acceptance and forgiveness will help you heal and sets us free. Say these words and be healed. The past is forgiven. You have the key; just unlock the chain. You are free. It is the only way to be free, find peace and happiness. It is a choice.

"I can forgive, but I cannot forget, is only another way of saying, I cannot forgive."

– Henry Ward Beecher

I believe that being able to deal with the sudden changes of life makes you a survivor, which defines your human spirit and soul. What are most important in life are your beliefs, since they have everything to do with how you live. By learning from your experiences, you will be able to have peace and happiness in your life. Forget about whom you were; accept who you are, and who you can be.

Elements Found in Happiness

Life
Free will
Hope
"Your soul" – "your very essence"
Dominion over other species
Sustenance
Gratification
Shelter
Love
Friendship
Creativity
Passion
Destiny

Facts of Life

It is a fact, that it is important how to act. That a little bit of this, and a little bit of that; makes a lot of what makes your life to be where it is at. Your life could be a bunch of crap where you may have been at; but you placed your order for that. You chose to accept the crap and your attitude on how to act.

Your attitude and how you react can dictate the facts that get to where you are at. You may not know that to be a fact. It may take a lifetime to discover that people do not scar or give you pain that throws you to the mat. It is your acceptance of their mistreatment that knocks you off track.

The thorn in your arm that could have been self-inflicted will do you no harm if you know the right facts. Every road has its own thorn that can hold you back from the way you react. It has always been your decision to accept the hurt and the scars that prevent you from being able to heal from all the attacks.

Now you know that life's happiness is all about your decision on how you react. It is never too late to take this road with thorns called life to where you want to be at. We are all human, be comfortable with this fact.

You can either allow your experiences to destroy you or redefine you. How you view your life will help you to survive. It takes courage to be able to deal with life's sudden changes. Sticks and stones may break your bones but you will decide if the words and names will ever hurt you.

How can an awakening do you harm unless you have not awoken? We are all much stronger than we initially think when something bad happens in our life. We all have free will that allows us to move forward by overcoming our self-pity. No one can defeat you. You can only defeat yourself. And that is a choice.

"It is never too late to become what you might have become."

– George Eliot

Faith, Hope, Belief, Logic, and Knowledge

The most important decision you will make in your life is what you choose for your beliefs since they have everything to do with how you live. Faith, Hope, and Belief are possibly the three important fabrics that keep most people's lives together, enough to survive the lessons we need to learn. Combining Logic and Knowledge with faith, hope, and belief requires the retention of your free will that enables you to become more human.

It takes courage to be able to deal with life's sudden changes. You may not fully recover but you can adapt. The battle is often won by finding a source of hope that will push you forward. To travel with hope is more important than arriving at your destination. A dream not yet realized offers far more benefits than the reality one faces when they give up hope. Never give up hope, for without hope, food and water will not be enough to nourish your body, mind, and soul. No one can defeat you. You can only defeat yourself.

Believing that creator will provide does not happen unless you work hard to get what you want. Hoping for a miracle is the same as hoping to win the lottery or hoping to receive an entitlement. Hoping for an entitlement is not what President Franklin Delano Roosevelt meant during his "Four Freedoms Speech" in his State of the Union Address on January 6, 1941: "The freedom of speech, the freedom of worship, the freedom from want, and the freedom from fear…" "Freedom from want," means you have the responsibility to provide for your own needs and the free will to pursue the occupation of your choice. Often "freedom of want" is achieved with stable and enduring relationships, education, hard work, sacrifice, and by saving a portion of your earnings. The Creator rewards those who believe in their ability to help themselves with an honest day's work. That is the difference between having hope and hoping.

Faith, Hope, and Belief are embodied in most religions of humankind. With these important fabrics rewoven into my life, I was able to walk the path and create a track to run on and the rest is history. From the fruits of my efforts, I would like to give back the Faith, Hope, Belief, Logic and Knowledge to all the good people that helped me and others like me who need a path to walk on and then a track to run on.

Humans have become more logical, facts build our knowledge and belief system. A logical person gathers facts and does not rely on faith alone. No one should resolutely affect your pursuit of the truth. We are gravitating towards building a belief system that is constructed mainly on materials based on facts.

"Logic and knowledge are imperative to the formation of a healthy, balanced, and constructive belief system. The very essence of intelligence clings to the foundations formed by a belief system relying on facts as opposed to hearsay and speculation. The progress humanity makes can always attribute its strides to the idea that human beings are lucky to have been blessed with intelligence and integrity, especially compared to other organisms that we share the planet Earth with. Deductive reasoning is a crucial tool that pertains to the intelligence and intellectualism of the human race and ultimately contributes to the good and progress of humanity. One must always be vigilant and alert for the possibility of being conned into believing generalized conclusions based on speculation rather than fact."

– Garrett Foster

"He who has health, has hope. And he who has hope, has everything."

– Old Arabian Proverb and credit has also been given to Thomas Carlyle

----

"For when I am powerless, it is then that I am strong."

– Paul, the Apostle 2 Corinthians 12:10, King James Version (KJV)

"We are taught to nurture the health of our body, mind, and soul; often they are neglected. While our health declines as each year passes, we value our soul more knowing that it is all that will remain."

– Brian Michael Good

RESET: CONTROL, ALT, DELETE

Acceptance is a Gift

How you view yourself should be far more important than what others think of you. Accepting yourself the way you are is the best gift you can give yourself. You are much better than you think you are.

Acceptance helps you to skip forward and live in the present. Sometimes you meet someone and you can skip forward because of the greeting, the acceptance, and the goodbye. Waiting was the hardest part and finally, one person and the acceptance among strangers pushed me over the fence totally into the present. Say hello to a stranger. They will greet you with a smile almost every time. Everyone needs a chance to be fulfilled with acceptance, which is the impetus to heal old wounds.

When you meet another person or when two or more are gathered you will have the opportunity to create the gift of acceptance, the epitome of what humanity should be! The higher you raise yourself in the better treatment of others, the better view you will have of the future.

Often respect is like seeing your reflection while looking at the surface of still water.

"Respect, like your reflection, must be projected first (good manners) in order to see the same reflection of respect returned."

– Brian Michael Good

"I have just three things to teach: simplicity, patience, compassion. These three are your greatest treasures."

– Lao Tzu

"Health is the greatest gift, contentment the greatest wealth, faithfulness the best relationship."

– Buddha

"God's gift to us is the gift of life and your gift to God is what you do with your life."

– Joe Langton

"Everything we take for granted is a gift; most of us only realize its value upon its loss."

– Brian Michael Good

Fear, Anxiety, Anger, and Depression

Just be fearless. Like me and others like me. Like firefighters, law enforcement, military men and women, astronauts, deep sea fishermen, cave explorers, miners, lumberjacks, skyscraper workers, surgeons, bullfighters, hi-rise window washers, EMTs, race car drivers, single mothers, cowboys-cowgirls, athletes, skydivers, airplane pilots, school bus drivers, and truck drivers especially in Alaska and northern climates.

"If you suffer from Fear, Anxiety, Anger, or Depression you may be picking up people's feelings and emotions. You might be an Empath."

– www.EmpathGuide.com

"How to Know if You Are an Empath"

www.WikiHow.com/Know-if-You-Are-an-Empath

Depression is like a rip tide current that never ends. If you try to swim back to shore, your efforts will be futile and it will only tire you out and make it that much more difficult for you to survive. To escape depression, just like the rip tide current, you need to swim sideways or seek help by allowing a lifeguard... 800-273-TALK (8255) or medicine carry you to calmer waters.

When you remember the past too much you don't heal; this can lead to depression. When you try to view the future too much, it can cause anxiety and fear. But when you live in the now, it makes you right, glad to be living in the moment. So it's time to deal with your life with a positive approach one day at a time and create new memories. Yes, you can replace old memories with new ones and start over in the present. I find that the best place to live is in the now.

There will never be enough breath in your lungs to sustain the depths of your despair; just like the depths of the ocean that cannot be sustained indefinitely without being resupplied with fresh air. In both cases you will not survive unless you take the necessary action needed before your final breath... Come up for air by going for a walk and just breathe.

Some of us compromise with our fear, some of us adapt to our fear, some of us are consumed by our fear, some of us are defeated by our fear, and some of us overcome our fear. Confronting fear is an instinctive response for survival. To be held captive by fear in any form is always a choice.

If you are a survivor, like me and others like me, you will not be held captive by fear, anger, hatred, anxiety or depression. Just be fearless. It might be the only way to save yourself from fear. Fear can consume you and spit you out dead. Feeling paralyzed with fear is not an option. Fear decreases in exact proportion to your increase in hope. Love heals and forgiveness removes fear. Forgiving others who have hurt you will help you heal.

Choose to live through your hurricanes of life. Some of the most talented, successful, and famous people in the world have done well in life even though they have suffered from depression, suicidal thoughts, and survived abuse. Just be fearless. Individuals in numerous occupations do it every day.

"You gain strength, courage and confidence by every experience in which you really stop to look fear in the face. You are able to say to yourself, 'I have lived through this horror. I can take the next thing that comes along.' You must do the thing you think you cannot do."

– Eleanor Roosevelt, First Lady, Diplomat, Human Rights Activist

----

"Fear not. Never look back, never give up, never stop trying, never quit, not even a bit."

– Brian Michael Good

"Courage is not the absence of fear, but rather the judgement that something else is more important than fear."

– Ambrose Redmoon

"Fear decreases in exact proportion to your increase in hope."

– Brian Michael Good

"For when I am powerless, it is then that I am strong."

– Paul, the Apostle

"We have nothing to fear but fear itself."

– Franklin D Roosevelt

"Life's journey often requires great courage to overcome our greatest fears."

– Brian Michael Good

"Courage is resistance to fear, mastery of fear not absence of fear."

– Mark Twain

"Rather than listening to the person with anger in their voice, empower yourself by listening to your inner voice of reason."

– Brian Michael Good

"Fear is what stops you… courage is what keeps you going."

– Unknown author

"Fear is a choice. Feeling paralyzed with fear is not an option. Just be fearless. It might be the only way to save yourself from fear. Fear can consume you and spit you out dead."

– Brian Michael Good

"Anger, hatred, fear, is very bad for our health"

– Dalai Lama

"You are chained by your decision to accept the fear, scars, and pain that you allowed others to bestow on you. It was your acceptance of their mistreatment that stops you from being able to heal from all the attacks. You have the key once you discover that the fear, scars, and pain were self-inflicted. Just unlock your chains. That is a choice."

– Brian Michael Good

"Holding on to anger is like grasping a hot coal with the intent of throwing it at someone else; you are the one who gets burned."

– Buddha

"Forgiving is not forgetting; it's actually remembering by not becoming an abuser; by using your free will not to hit back with anger or revenge. It's an opportunity for a new beginning, a second chance, a learning experience by not allowing anyone to hurt or abuse you again."

– Brian Michael Good

Healing Yourself

Your life can change without notice; in just seconds that could change your life's course forever… only if you let it. Nearly everything can be fixed. That is a choice. Only you can choose to heal yourself. Let today be the first day of your new existence.

A scar only reminds us of the past. Sometimes a scar is an invisible wound that was not mended and never healed. When you accept that people do not scar or give you pain; you will realize that your open wound was self-inflicted. It is your acceptance of other's mistreatment that stops the open wound from being healed that prevents you from moving past the hurt that only you view as a scar no matter how fresh or old the wound.

You no longer need to feel the bitterness towards your parents, friends, or family since you allowed that pain to be inflicted onto you because you chose to accept the hurt. Only you can choose to heal yourself by working on your pain, hang ups, and hurts by forgiving the people that you think affected your life in a negative way. It is the only way to be free, attain, and find peace. Remove all your fears by solving your problems. I now grow stronger each day without fear.

Start a new journey filled with the passion and the love and forgiveness that you deserve. When you forgive… you will have made the decision to move forward. Only you can heal yourself. It is a choice.

You are chained by your decision to accept the fear, scars, and pain that you allowed others to bestow on you. It was your acceptance of their mistreatment that stops you from being able to heal from all the attacks. You have the key once you discover that the fear, scars, and pain were self-inflicted. Just unlock your chains. Forgiveness removes fear. Forgiving others who have hurt you will help you heal. How you view your life will help you to survive.

Life's experiences are not woven with a constant thread; Life in our world is constantly changing. We must repurpose what we have endured and the lessons we have learned; creating a renewed sense of hope. Life is what it is. The question is: what are you willing to do to change your life?

Changes or events that happen in your life can be fixed or healed with a positive mental attitude. But when your life is over; it never comes back and you'll never know you could have made it to where you once thought was impossible. Most people that have had suicidal thoughts do change their minds and later in life think, "What was I thinking? I almost gave up my life."

Challenges, hardships and obstacles are part of what life's journey is all about. You are not always in control of what happens to you, but you are in control how you react to it. You can allow your experiences to destroy you or redefine you. A person who navigates life's challenges, hardships, and obstacles with stern resolve is able to sail in all winds. How you view your life will help you to survive. No one can defeat you. You can only defeat yourself. It takes courage to be able to deal with life's sudden changes. If you face your challenges, hardships, and obstacles with a positive mental attitude, you will find that it takes half the effort to overcome them. The sum of your challenges, hardships, and obstacles will define your human spirit and can become your strength.

Rejoice about your decision to release the chains of your pain and scars that you allowed others to bestow on you. People do not scar or give you pain. It is your acceptance of other's mistreatment that allows the continuance of your mistreatment. Do not allow this to happen. Walk away. Everything is in your control.

It is your own fault if you listen to the naysayers. There is one exception; it is hard to walk away from your parents when you live under their roof.

Before my failed suicide attempt on October 23, 2003 I accepted the abuse that I allowed others to bestow upon me. I blame no one but "me" for not allowing myself to heal, especially as I became an adult, when I kept the hurt and I didn't seek help.

It took me a lifetime to discover that people do not scar you or give you pain; it was my acceptance of their mistreatment.

I used to blame others for every hurt and the scars, from the years of abuse (emotionally, physically, and mentally) during my childhood and teenage years, but now, having forgiven them (my abusers) for everything I realize the abuse was self-inflicted. It was my acceptance of their mistreatment. I blame myself for not being able to heal from the hurt and the scars.

I found that self-pity was one of my greatest weaknesses. Self-pity doesn't do anyone any good. We are all much stronger than we initially think when something bad happens in our life.

Now, I walk away from abuse. If you are a survivor like me and others like me, you will not be held captive by fear, anxiety, anger, or depression. Just be fearless. It might be the only way to save yourself from fear. Fear can consume you and spit you out dead. Feeling paralyzed with fear is not an option. Love heals and forgiveness removes fear. Forgiving others who have hurt you will help you heal.

You must change your perspective by infusing new activities into your life. If you care about others you will care less about life's problems. It takes time to change your perspective. It took many years for these pearls of wisdom to wash ashore as a result of my hurricanes and it took even more time for the lessons expressed in passages above to be fully absorbed into the new me.

What I have learned from my personal experience can give you hope. It is my hope that you and others know. You are not Alone or Forgotten. Your life will improve. Peace and happiness are renewed for those who seek it. I believe that you too will find wisdom in the pearls that have washed ashore as a result of my hurricanes and count yourself a survivor.

"The ability to be in the present moment is a major component of mental wellness."

– Abraham Maslow

"The concept of total wellness recognizes that our every thought, word, and behavior affects our greater health and well-being. And we, in turn, are affected not only emotionally but also physically and spiritually."

– Greg Anderson

"I have come to realize that without the engine; the body, getting a tune-up; the driver, the mind, cannot get where it wants to go in life very well. A healthy mind begins with a healthy body and vice versa."

– Brian Michael Good

"Sticks and stones may break your bones but you will decide if the words and names will ever hurt you."

– Brian Michael Good

"Time heals all wounds."

– Unknown author

"When you speak of a negative or hear a negative from someone that you choose not to accept. Just say the words "cancel – clear"."

– Donna Marie Wright

Coping Skills

Get enough sleep
Go for a walk – Get some sunlight
Develop New Friendships
Watch your diet
Change your daily routine
Play some good music and chill for awhile
Develop a way to clear your head…
Just say the words "cancel – clear"
Exercise
Forgive Others
Spiritualize
Meditate
Journal
Set Limits
Visualize
Set Goals

> "No one can defeat you. You can only defeat yourself. No one can truly save you. You must save yourself."
>
> – Brian Michael Good

The wisdom in our future is discovered in the present. You cannot go forward unless you let go of the past. Reset: You are in CONTROL, Change your Perspective ALT, Forget the past. DELETE>.

Saying... BYBF be your best friend. Me, myself, and I are my best friends. I can count on Me most of the time. I have learned life's lessons the hard way from the error of my ways. When you graduate high school or college, you may have made your last friend except if you have the opportunity to make a friend at work or with your partner. But you always have yourself.

Thoughts are like building blocks. Put enough thoughts together and an idea will take shape. When your idea develops, you will often come up with a solution to a problem.

> "Talking to yourself once in a blue moon is acceptable. Arguing with yourself is not acceptable. So, why are you still in denial?"
>
> – Brian Michael Good

> "Develop a way to clear your head... Just say a positive phrase silently or out loud by repeating it to yourself until it clears your head."
>
> – Brian Michael Good

"Songs will never grow old when they are done by great performers. Play some good music and enjoy a comfortable chill by listening to your favorite music. A great coping skill."

– Brian Michael Good

"Help someone in need with kindness including yourself."

– Brian Michael Good

"No one can defeat you. You can only defeat yourself. No one can truly save you. You must save yourself."

– Brian Michael Good

"Acceptance – Let go of the past to get ahead in the present."

– Brian Michael Good

"Do not dwell on problems in which you cannot effect any change."

– Brian Michael Good

Getting a Tune-Up

My fourth pearl washed ashore from a fourth hurricane that started on June 12, 2009. It was something I had to learn the hard way. I was deeply depressed for several months. I faced my depression, challenges and fears and decided I would not be held captive. When I fully made this decision, my depression was gone.

You burn more calories when you are more positive, with each step you burn off the negative emotions. I feel so good when I go out and exercise. I feel good when I create a new passion. I wish everyone feels as good as me. I don't live with depression. Depression lives with me. I don't give depression that much power. You can decide to lift yourself up and do something positive in your life.

Seven out of ten adults do not exercise regularly. I found that working out at the gym at least three days or more a week has increased my ability to implement change in my life. I have come to realize that without the engine, the body, getting a tune-up, and the driver, the mind, cannot get where it wants to go in life very well. A healthy mind begins with a healthy body and vice versa. The mind thinks so much more clearly when the body gets a tune-up at least three days a week. Dealing with life's challenges has much to do with your body getting a tune up.

Watching my diet by eating food using dietary guidelines with USDA suggested nutritional value and maintaining a healthy gut were major steps forward in my recovery from depression. Kefir, kimchi, kombucha, miso, natto, sauerkraut, and tempeh are fermented probiotic foods for a healthy gut. I stopped eating foods with artificial flavors and colors. I gave up fast food, frozen and other processed food; food with ingredients I didn't understand. This step forced me to cook my own balanced meals with ninety percent organic and natural ingredients. Instead of soft drinks, diet soda, sports drinks and fruit juices with high-fructose corn syrup, sugar substitutes, preservatives and other ingredients, I drank water and green tea unsweetened. I got used to it fairly quickly with a positive attitude. I ate more vegetables and fruits instead of brownies and cakes. I allowed myself to have a daily cup of coffee with half a teaspoon of organic sugar, fruit juices with no added sugar diluted with water, and alcohol occasionally.

Three foods are linked with depression and possibly other forms illnesses: refined grains (foods made with white flour, enriched wheat flour or all-purpose flour), soft drinks, and fast food. According to a 2012 study in the journal Public Health Nutrition, people who eat fast food are 51 percent more likely to develop depression than those who don't. This includes commercial baked goods, hamburgers, hot dogs and pizza.1

"The cells in your body are surrounded by mostly water… and there is a mountain of evidence which proves that the type of water you drink is the most important element of your health, because it changes how the cells absorb the nutrients, and how they behave."

– Kacper Postawski, Author

There is always a possibility of a storm on the horizon. Hurricanes will always be a possibility so be ready to deal with life's sudden changes. As a survivor, living in the present with hope and a positive mental attitude will be always be how I stay in the eye of my hurricane; safe from the storm around me. Because varied combinations of challenges, hardships and obstacles make up every life.

I hope that you too will find wisdom in these pearls that have washed ashore as a result of my hurricanes and count yourself a survivor. The hurricanes keep coming; I gain strength with each pearl of wisdom. We are all human, be happy with this fact.

"A lot of what passes for depression these days is nothing more than a body saying that it needs work."

– Geoffrey Norman

"The concept of total wellness recognizes that our every thought, word, and behavior affects our greater health and well-being. And we, in turn, are affected not only emotionally but also physically and spiritually."

– Greg Anderson

"To wish to be well is a part of becoming well."

– Seneca (5 BC – 65 AD)

"Knowing is not enough; we must apply. Willing is not enough; we must do."

– Johann Wolfgang von Goethe

----

[1] "3 Foods Linked with Depression," by Deborah Enos, Live Science. www.LiveScience.com/41759-foods-linked-with-depression.html

Change

You should effect change when it comes to your mental, physical, emotional, or spiritual health. I know my daughter did this over twelve years ago when I experienced the most self-destructive part of my life. I no longer blame Amelia for her absence. I failed to give her a good role model as a parent as I should have during parts of my parenting. I fought with my spouse in front of her, swearing with anger just like what I learned from my father. Do not make my mistake; I placed work ahead of quality time that I could have spent with my daughter Amelia.

My daughter, Amelia, and I met for dinner on September 24, 2007 just before I moved to Florida on October 1, 2007. Amelia called me in June 2008 asking if she could come down to Florida and see me but plans can change from week to week. She lost her ride down to Florida and I lost my dream.

The wisdom in our future is discovered in the present. You cannot go forward unless you let go of the past. Reset: You are in CONTROL, Change your Perspective ALT, Forget the past. DELETE>. We all have the power within us to change and survive.

Plan a change. Do something different in your life — move out of your comfort zone. What is most important is the foundation, a step by step outline of your plan that will encourage you to do something different outside your comfort zone. Your plan will likely fail without a step by step outline, the change may not happen if you don't plan or follow through with your plan to venture out of your comfort zone.

If a rabbit is chased by a fox in the woods, the rabbit goes down its hole and always has a backup plan, another exit to escape. If the fox knows where the rabbit lives, the rabbit digs another hole and makes a new home, a new life. The rabbit doesn't stay in the past. The rabbit is always working towards the future. Humans were like the animal kingdom until we moved to cities. We just became secure and maybe lazy because life got too easy. Build a new and better life. I did.

"The clock's ticking… The longer you wait to change your life the harder it becomes to implement change. Sixty years old is mid-life if you consider that a healthy person with modern medical care might live to one hundred twenty. So what are you waiting for?"

– Brian Michael Good

"I cannot say whether things will get better if we change; what I can say is they must change if they are to get better."

– G. C. Lichtenberg

"It has been said that in a lifetime we live many lives. If you don't like your life begin your next life within your present life by implementing change."

– Brian Michael Good

Solving Your Problems

"Mind over matter. If it matters, you will put your mind to it. The mind is capable of solving anything that matters."

– Brian Michael Good

"Whatever the mind can conceive and believe, the mind can achieve with PMA. (Positive Mental Attitude)"

– W. Clement Stone

If you have a problem, then do everything you can to correct or rectify this problem. Do not dwell on problems in which you cannot effect any change. You cannot change the negatives of the past. You can effect change in the present. Dwelling on negatives affects our rhythm and holds us back from the present. The future may be viewed and anticipated but it is not laid out precisely like a blueprint. We can choose to steer off course or amend it. We have choices. You have free will. We need to Reset our perspective in layers. We need to Reset our acceptance and understanding. We do not change overnight. Change one day at a time. Reset from the inside out.

"Do what you can where you are with what you have."

— Theodore Roosevelt

"Now is no time to think of what you do not have. Think of what you can do with what there is."

— Ernest Hemingway

"Strength does not come from physical capacity. It comes from an indomitable will."

— Mahatma Gandhi

"If you do not try to change your world, your world will change you."

— Brian Michael Good

"Do not dwell on problems in which you cannot effect any change."

— Brian Michael Good

Control the Present

Only you can improve the way you view yourself and how you are perceived by others. You can affect change in your self-esteem and improve the way you view yourself with a positive mental attitude. Your attitude affects your self-esteem and how you are viewed by others.

I grow stronger every day knowing I am in control of the direction of my life. The sum of your challenges, hardships, and obstacles can become your strength. You can effect change in the present. You will not to be held captive by fear, anxiety or depression. Be a survivor. That is a choice.

Most of us live our lives in the proactive, reactive, or passive mode. When you are proactive, you tend to be positive and to be prepared for what could happen. When you are reactive, you tend to respond when something has already happened. A proactive approach can result in a better opportunity for control and fulfillment; whereas the reactive mode can result in stress, which can make any problem even more difficult to solve and may lead to failure.

Just like water, wind, waves, and ice are the erosion agents of our beaches that bring change to our shorelines. Fear, anxiety, and depression are the erosion agents of our hope that bring changes to our mental, physical, emotional, or spiritual health. It is important to know where you are, so you can adjust the direction of your life in a positive direction.

"All we can really do or control is living in the moment."

– Brian Michael Good

"The ability to be in the present moment is a major component of mental wellness."

– Abraham Maslow

"Fear, anxiety, and depression decreases in exact proportion to your increase in hope."

– Brian Michael Good

"Every endeavor in life is not about the odds of success but about your passion, your belief, and your indomitable will."

– Brian Michael Good

"Because a fellow has failed once or twice or a dozen times, you don't want to set him down as a failure till he's dead or loses his courage."

– George Horace Lorimer

"The secret of getting ahead is getting started."

– Mark Twain

"Strive for progress, not perfection."

– Unknown author

\-

Living in the Present

Live in the present, where it is the best place to live. Immediately clear any negative thoughts before it turns into fear. Do not dwell on a negative. Throw it out of you, skip forward. Do a different activity right away and think of a positive situation.

"Develop a way to clear your head… Just say a positive phrase silently or out loud by repeating it to yourself until it clears your head."

– Brian Michael Good

Live in the present so you can affect the future. If I can make it happen, (then) so can you. We are humans; negatives will tend to pop up from time to time. If you can feel pain living in the past, forgiving others will help you move into the present.

When you remember the past too much, you don't heal and this can lead to depression. When you try to view the future too much, it can cause anxiety. But when you live in the Now, it makes you feel right; glad to be living in the moment.

You will not to be held captive by fear, anxiety, or depression. Develop a way to clear your head. Just say "cancel – clear".

How you manage your expectations is the secret to happiness and finding peace in your life. One perspective at a time. Happiness and peace are for those who seek it. You are not alone and you are not forgotten. Your life will improve. Take control of your life and be a survivor. Talk to someone who cares. Call 800-273-TALK (8255). It is your choice.

"Your thoughts create your experience. Your experience creates your reality. Everything you say is a projection and a creation. If it is not a loving thought, then it is a fearful thought. Say what you want to do. Say what is in your heart. The words you use have power. You are always placing an order with every word you speak. It is the journey that is most important part of our life. Forgiveness is the key. Forgiving others sets us free. Focus on loving yourself."

– Jodi Cardoza

"You are chained by your decision to accept the fear, scars, and pain that you allowed others to bestow on you. It was your acceptance of their mistreatment that stops you from being able to heal from all the attacks. You have the key once you discover that the fear, scars, and pain were self-inflected. Just unlock your chains. It is a choice."

– Brian Michael Good

"Do not dwell in the past, do not dream of the future, concentrate the mind on the present moment."

– Buddha

"You are chained by your decision to accept the fear, scars, and pain that you allowed others to bestow on you. It was your acceptance of their mistreatment that stops you from being able to heal from all the attacks. You have the key once you discover that the fear, scars, and pain were self-inflected. Just unlock your chains. It is a choice."

– Brian Michael Good

"Do not dwell in the past, do not dream of the future, concentrate the mind on the present moment."

– Buddha

Rebuilding Your Life

We can lose everything and still rebuild our Life. Your life is full of choices. We are chained by the negatives of society, fears of the future or our past! We have all been given a key. Just unlock your chain. You can effect change in the present. In the Now!

I have "Been There" many, many times. "Being There" is no excuse for "Staying There." Free will is our greatest gift after life itself, that being said, free will must be exercised wisely.

Choose to begin to change one day at a time; tiny steps where you position yourself in steady motion of happiness and tranquility instead of allowing yourself to be hashed around beyond your control. You have more control than you think.

Everything is definitely in your control except the laws of nature. It is how you react to it that is in your control. Every time you step in a more positive direction it's like building muscle in your body.

People need to take small steps, one at a time. Create a new life from what is left of the former life. What you do differently this week will help you go from the old to the new you.

Take a minute… Ask yourself what will make me happy. For most people something dramatic has to happen from your life's experience to teach you to walk the right path.

How we are raised sets into motion our vibration within society. Everything vibrates. The colors of nature are very important to be viewed each day.

Break the cycle. Watch less news. Create your own world of good and happiness.

Listen to different types of music. Find what type of music makes you the most happy. Go to a library and listen for free. All over the world everyone is touched by music.

It is extremely important to listen to the right music every day.

Some music or programs will make you depressed; avoid them at all cost. What you choose to watch on TV will influence your life more than you ever realize.

Readiness. Right, Reaction. What you say does make a difference. Definitely your values have much to do with accomplishing your goals and fulfilling your potential.

Rationalize the way you think. Change your belief system. Important to learn to forgive and let go of the past. It is gone. Your willingness to change is the first step.

I decided thirteen years ago to break the cycle from one generation to the next. I completed fifty percent of an abuse course in 2002 (It was my choice, it wasn't court ordered). In 2005 I passed an anger management course. These self-help programs helped me to become more human. I have been divorced for over eleven years and I am finally comfortable and happy being alone. Time is quick; it catches up to all of us. I will live my life over again. I am ready to make new friendships, a family, and maybe children. Life has become a real slice of heaven for me these days,

You must strive to act as the person you would like to become, as an actor would become the persona of the character of a play or movie. It takes at least thirteen weeks before you transition into a new person. You must believe that you are the "new you" before other people perceive "you" as this "new you".

Over the course of thirteen weeks you will begin to believe and trust that your success is just around the corner. People start to perceive you to be more successful. Live life in the present, in the now and it will happen.

If I can get up after my near-fatal suicide attempt and physically, mentally, emotionally, and spiritually become more functional and then take the ball over the goal line, then why can't you do the same.

Take small steps, one at a time; creating a new life from what is left of how you chose to live before. What you do differently each day will help you go from the old to the new you. Take a minute... Ask yourself "what will make me happy?" For most people it takes a dramatic chain of events to unfold and it seems to happen all at once yet it happens over many months. We need to go through change in order for us to walk the right path. Choose to begin to change one day at a time, tiny steps where you position yourself in a steady motion of happiness and tranquility instead of allowing yourself to be hashed around beyond your control.

Train yourself to think these thoughts, "I have free will. It is my choice." I suggest that if put a new plan into action and stay with this new attitude about how you might choose to view and live your life; you will positively have more happy moments than ever before in your lifetime.

"Think of this motto before you react or respond to any situation: Readiness, Right, Reaction."

– Brian Michael Good

Find Someone Who Cares

Drowning

During the summer of my tenth birthday, my older brother and I went swimming at the Quincy, Massachusetts quarry. I started to drown as I went under water for the third time.

A fifteen old boy jumped in and pulled me out as I went under. What I felt could've been the last time. He cared and saved my life. Find and talk to someone who cares.

"There is nothing on this earth more to be prized than true friendship."

– Thomas Aquinas

Skydiving

During my twenties, I had four parachute malfunctions out of one hundred forty-seven jumps (C-18640 License, USPA). Every skydiver wears two parachutes when they jump. The main parachute is the first parachute the skydiver attempts to deploy. The second parachute is called the reserve parachute. Approximately one in a thousand deployments of a main parachute results in a malfunction in which the main must be cut away by pulling a handle that also deploys the reserve after the main is severed. My malfunction rate was 20 times the normal rate. Am I blessed or what!

One of my four malfunctions was when my Automatic Activation Device deployed at 6500 feet instead of 1000 feet. We were doing a four way diamond off the wing strut and step of a Cessna 182 at 7500 feet. The diamond relative work was unstable from the moment we left the plane. The Automatic Activation Device deployed my pilot chute on the top of my reserve parachute at 6500 feet by accident, 1000 feet into the jump. The pilot chute just lay on top of my back as if no air could take it for 1.5 seconds. Enough time for the other three skydivers to notice that my pilot chute was about catch air and deploy my reserve parachute prematurely, fortunate for all of us…

If one of the skydivers was directly over me as my reserve parachute deployed, we both probably would have died. The skydiver over me would have been traveling at 120 miles per hour and when my reserve deployed, my descent would have slowed to fifteen miles an hour. Thus, a possible impact between two skydivers at one hundred miles an hour, the impact would have resulted in our deaths.

Each time I faced death; I knew I wanted to live. The licensed rigger who packed and inspected my emergency parachute was someone who cared because he knew that the reserve parachute had to work in order to save my life. He cared and saved my life. Find and talk to someone who cares.

Finding Your Destiny

    Finding your destiny has much to do with finding out what makes you happy. You need to take the necessary steps to put your life on the right course to find your passion. Choose a passion you enjoy doing; so even if you do not meet your destiny, you will be happy with your life. Always have a backup plan. You may find that your hobby is the passion that becomes your destiny. We should value the passion we have for our life's work more than we value material gain. Every endeavor in life is not about the odds of success but about your belief, your passion, and your indomitable will. Never let your attitude be the reason for your failure. The only thing you will truly regret in your life is who you could have been. Life will always be what you make of it. Forget about whom you were; accept who you are, and who you can be.

    If you have not developed a passion, a concept, or a theme for your life on how best to live, you will never know you could have made it to a place you once thought was impossible. I ask you to develop a theme or a concept about what you enjoy the most in your life. Write it down and let others know about it. Never put your destiny in the hands of a naysayer, do not listen to them.

"If you never venture out of your comfort zone and put your idea into action, another person surely will."

– Brian Michael Good

RESET: CONTROL, ALT, DELETE

Seven out of ten people do not enjoy their vocation. Most of the time people find their first couple of jobs by circumstance or chance rather than creating a plan based on their passion.

Getting a college degree or working in a trade may increase your income potential substantially over a person with a high school degree through the course of your career. However, a college degree is no longer a guarantee to get a job right out of college. Many college graduates wait years to get their first professional job. I was a professional recruiter for thirteen years. The rule of thumb is that it takes forty hours a week of effort every week to get a job. Be prepared to handle the rejection you will receive with a positive mental attitude in order to get that first professional job. A positive attitude influences our behavior and dictates a successful approach. Remember, you are much better than you think you are.

I did not start college until I was twenty years old. I graduated college when I was almost twenty-seven years old and sold insurance for the first three years after college before I found my career as recruiter. I was thirty years old when I started my first career job.

Failures are stepping-stones to success and your destiny. Failure allows you to reinvent yourself. You learn more from your mistakes and failures than from any degree of success. Success can only be grasped for a moment before it becomes a distant oasis not to be found again unless you thirst for the knowledge found in the well fed by your mistakes and failures.

"The costs to society are much less to feed an open mind with a school meal than to feed a closed mind that no longer has the appetite to believe in the American Dream."

– Brian Michael Good

The pursuit of the American Dream is alive but not well and may seem obscure and improbable for most of us since is it is harder than ever to achieve with such an abundance of low paying jobs; but the truth is the American Dream has never been easy to attain. Yet, the elusive American Dream is still achievable for anyone with the right attitude, buying behavior, education, savings, knowing the value of hard work, and indomitable will.

Let us not mourn the passing of the American Dream just because we have given up hope; many of us are left hoping to win the lottery. Anyone living near or below the poverty line knows very well that the higher cost of services essential for daily survival is a formidable goal for them. Still, many Americans take these blessings for granted.

The American Dream is even more elusive for America's hungry children who need the creation of a national Smart Start Nutrition Program that would provide two nutritious meals, breakfast and lunch, at school to all pupils in compulsory education regardless of their ability to pay.

Think about a car not having ample petro/gas start the engine, as the body not getting the proper nutrition, preventing the driver from arriving at their desired destination, an engaged mind likewise cannot develop the knowledge base on life skills that will be needed to achieve upward mobility.

Smart Start Nutrition would be the first step in providing an equal educational opportunity that would have a direct correlation to a decrease in the need for public assistance and additional prison space twenty years later.

The pursuit of the American Dream is alive but not well and may seem obscure and improbable for most of us since is it is harder than ever to achieve with such an abundance of low paying jobs; but the truth is the American Dream has never been easy to attain. Yet, the elusive American Dream is still achievable for anyone with the right attitude, buying behavior, education, savings, knowing the value of hard work, and indomitable will.

Only Sweden, Finland and Estonia provide free school meals to all pupils in compulsory education regardless of their ability to pay.

"It is easier to build strong children than to repair broken men."

– Frederick Douglass

Find a purpose for your life and you will do extraordinary things. You are in the center of your happiness when you pursue your passion. When you pursue your passion, you are the master of your environment. When you are the master of your environment, you often meet your destiny.

The pursuit of the American Dream is alive but not well and may seem obscure and improbable for most of us since is it is harder than ever to achieve with such an abundance of low paying jobs; but the truth is the American Dream has never been easy to attain. Yet, the elusive American Dream is still achievable with the right attitude, buying behavior, education, savings, and knowing the value of hard work.

People who are born and raised in America could learn many lessons of hope from their grandparents, great grandparents, and immigrants. The key to their success was their indomitable spirit to have stable and enduring relationships, educate themselves, hard work, sacrifice, and achieve higher savings rates.

I Wanted to Change the World

"When I was a young man, I wanted to change the world. I found it was difficult to change the world, so I tried to change my nation. When I found I couldn't change the nation, I began to focus on my town. I couldn't change the town and as an older man, I tried to change my family.

Now, as an old man, I realize the only thing I can change is myself, and suddenly I realize that if long ago I had changed myself, I could have made an impact on my family. My family and I could have made an impact on our town. Their impact could have changed the nation and I could indeed have changed the world."

– Unknown Monk, 1100 A.D.

"To be yourself in a world that is constantly trying to make you something else is the greatest accomplishment."

– Ralph Waldo Emerson

"You must be the change you want to see in the world."

– Mahatma Gandhi

"A great deal of talent is lost to the world for the want of a little courage."

– Sydney Smith

"To live is the rarest thing in the world. Most people exist, that is all."

– Oscar Wilde

Pearls of Wisdom: Life and Destiny

"Integrity, Honor, Trust, Loyalty, Respect, Reputation. These values should be nurtured as a mother cares for an infant. Without the proper attention, all of these values can be lost from one careless decision."

– Brian Michael Good

"Islam teaches that Destiny (nasib) is written with your own hands, then handed over to Creator, and He gives the judgement."

– Destiny (in Islam)? Religion Answers, Wiki

"If one advances confidently in the direction of his dreams, and endeavors to live the life which he has imagined, he will meet with a success unexpected in common hours."

– Henry David Thoreau

RESET: CONTROL, ALT, DELETE

"Mind over matter, if it matters, you will put your mind to it. The mind is capable of solving anything that matters."

– Brian Michael Good

"An invisible thread connects those who are destined to meet, regardless of time, place, and circumstance. The thread may stretch or tangle. But it will never break."

– Ancient Chinese Proverb

"Tomorrow is full of promise if you prepare for today."

– Brian Michael Good

"Be not afraid of greatness: some are born great, some achieve greatness, and some have greatness thrust upon them."

– William Shakespeare

"You often meet your destiny on the road you've taken to avoid it."

– Chinese proverb

"It is never too late to become what you might have become."

– George Eliot

"Great things come from people who are not afraid to risk making others around them feel uncomfortable with their futuristic vision."

– Brian Michael Good

"Watch your thoughts; they become words.
Watch your words; they become actions.
Watch your actions; they become habits.
Watch your habits; they become character.
Watch your character;
It becomes your destiny."

– Lao Tzu

"Don't be afraid of your fears. They are not there to scare you. They're there to let you know that something is worth it."

– C. JoyBell C., Author

"Every endeavor in life is not about the odds of success but about your belief, your passion, and your indomitable will."

– Brian Michael Good

Testicular Cancer

My first pearl washed ashore as result of my first hurricane. I had stage two testicular cancer. I was not aware of the warning signs of testicular cancer or and what I should have looked for. My first hurricane was not what I was planning as I was about to graduate college.

On my first day of awakening, I was told by my doctor that I had advanced testicular cancer. I had an active six pound tumor; a cancer between my abdomen and spine that was doubling every two months. We found it two months before it would have been too late for medical treatment. The cancer would have been twelve pounds two months after it was discovered and twenty-four pounds in four months. I had less than six months to live. It would have been too late for treatment if I had waited an additional two months to see a doctor. I had no health insurance while I was in college.

I am ninety-nine percent to the tenth degree cured of testicular cancer. The regime of chemotherapy for my cancer was just discovered in the previous year. My six-pound tumor had not spread throughout my body; it was localized between my abdomen and spine. My nurses and doctors were the best in world in my opinion.

My cancer, to some degree, changed my life. But humans tend to get back into the rat race and so did I.

When Doctor Hines told me I had cancer, my reply was, "I skydive almost every weekend and I face death with every jump; so, I will face my cancer the very same way, with a 'Positive Mental Attitude: PMA.'" – W. Clement Stone.

From October 1982 to March 6, 1983, I had an operation and four to five days in the hospital intensive chemotherapy treatments were scheduled. My cancer treatment was one of the two harshest chemotherapy regimens at the time. I lost all my hair in less than a week.

Three pounds of my tumor was gone after the first week of treatment. Why? Because of the Creator and I had PMA… a Positive Mental Attitude. The Creator gives you free will; you can give up or try to live.

In between my third and fourth chemotherapy treatment, I went to three weeks of insurance licensing training at Combined Insurance Company of America. This training gave me a path to walk on and kept my mind away from the worries of my demise. In February of 1983, I weighed one hundred and eight pounds with no hair, no beard and I looked like death warmed over.

I passed the insurance licensing and sales course and in the beginning of March of 1983, the day before I started my last five day chemotherapy treatment in the hospital at the New England Medical Center in Boston, Massachusetts.

Little did I know that my daughter Amelia would be born eight years later on the day I entered the hospital for my fourth and final treatment of chemotherapy.

I signed myself out of the hospital on the second day of my fourth and last five-day chemotherapy treatment. Everyone was upset at me. Dr. David Parkinson later said it was water under the bridge. Months later the doctors realized that I only needed three rounds of chemotherapy to be cured. This medical knowledge may not have been discovered as soon as it was if I had not checked myself out of the hospital prematurely.

Both of my hospital stays cost society over a million in today's dollars. Both times I was uninsured. I had to claim bankruptcy in 2004 and was approved for four credit cards in 2006 to early 2007.

Through my experiences, I have gathered many pearls of wisdom from my hurricanes. Without these pearls of wisdom, my hurricanes would have destroyed me.

Today, I will try to stay in the eye of my hurricane where I am safe from the storm around me. I will try to deal with my hurricanes and struggles in life with no blame or excuses. But my hurricanes keep coming. I gain strength with each pearl of wisdom that washes ashore.

Abuse is No Excuse

My childhood was filled with tension, excessive discipline, and yelling – at home and at grammar school – each contributed to a lower self-esteem and academic performance during my formative developmental years. Yelling and corporal punishment instilled fear in me. I carried such sentiments and emotional trauma with me into adulthood.

I was sexually abused as a teenager. I worked at a restaurant and the chef would grab my buttocks or penis as I was preparing a meal. It happened quite often during the several years I worked there. I saw him grab a waitress's buttocks on a daily basis and noticed that other cooks did the same. I thought that this was normal behavior for people that worked in restaurants. I did not know at the time that it was called sexual abuse.

In January 2003, I was homeless and stayed at a friend's house sleeping in her basement. One night as I was sleeping, her husband came home drunk and came downstairs and started to hit me with a baseball bat; telling me to leave. Fortunately, she heard him and came downstairs. My friend's husband then went outside and smashed my van's front windshield with the baseball bat. Her husband was arrested that night but, the damage was done. I got an apartment in April 2003. I faced homelessness six months later. This time I thought I had no one to turn to, so I decided to die by suicide.

It took a self-induced hurricane; my suicide attempt, when I did not heed the advice given to me to evacuate the coast (by properly dealing with personal issues including mental health, eviction, taxes, unemployment, and a failed marriage) which lead to three months of rehab for my twisted foot from my drug overdose, then eight months of homelessness. Ironically, these were the first steps to the road of recovery. Years later, I became a person who was kind, polite, giving, no anger, and grateful for all my blessings.

How did I accomplish this? By taking self-help programs and choosing to participate with a positive mental attitude. I had faced death several times and it did not change me until my near-fatal suicide attempt and recovery, it is my hope that *RESET Control, Alt, Delete* will show you the lessons I had to learn to gain back my self-respect. As I stated before, I started by taking an abuse course (not court ordered – my choice – you know – free will). After my suicide attempt I took and passed an anger management course. These self-help programs helped me to become a better person.

You must find a way to live even if you suffer from shunning, teasing, gossiping, bullying, shaming, child abuse, sexual abuse, verbal and/or physical abuse. You are the one who is responsible for your own life and the decisions you make.

"The evil in your life is the abuse you allow others to bestow on you. So, if you are a survivor like me and others like me, just be fearless. It might be the only way to save yourself from fear. Fear can consume you and spit you out dead."

– Brian Michael Good

"Find a man/woman/partner that will appreciate everything about you and won't try to change you or control your free will."

– Brian Michael Good

Death at My Door

I didn't expect to survive my suicide attempt. My near death experience should have killed me. But I should have read up on the statistics; four out of five suicide attempts fail.

In 2003, during a four week period, I lost my job, van and apartment; I spent four days in a county jail for not being able to pay child support. The Norfolk County Jail was filled to capacity so I was placed in the infirmary, on a cold floor and a dark room with a thin mattress and a light blanket. I was allowed to make one five-minute call a day. It was during this time, in that room, where I had my first thoughts of suicide. A psychologist once told me that that spending four days in jail under such conditions was enough to make me suicidal.

Tanya, my estranged wife told me she filed for divorce the evening I got out of county jail. The very next day, my landlord asked me to move out of my apartment in five days. I was deeply depressed. I saw no way out. There was nobody I could turn to for help and I did not know how to reach out to someone. Life no longer seemed worth living, Three days after I was released from the county jail and two days before my eviction, I attempted suicide. My near-fatal suicide attempt story began on October 23, 2003 when I overdosed on enough pills to kill an elephant, only to survive by a miracle that was the Creator's intervention. Was I brain dead before, or after, I overdosed on pills? Before I took my overdose of prescription drugs, I asked the Creator for forgiveness and help. I believed that death by suicide was an unforgivable act, it was wrong. I could have been created as a rock or tree but to be born as a human was the greatest gift by the Creator.

I was predestined to have a near death experience from my suicide attempt so I would care about suicide. The Creator knew I would write *Never Surrender Your Soul – your very essence, RESET: Control, Alt, Delete, and Quotes of Wisdom to Live By.*

Nearly everyone, at some time in his or her life, thinks about suicide. Some of the reasons why I attempted suicide included depression, unemployment, eviction and social pressures. A psychologist once told me that I had enough reasons but not to try it again. After a near-fatal suicide attempt, it is unlikely a person will ever try to attempt suicide again.

Tanya, my estranged wife, said that an EMT told her that I had thirty minutes to live without medical intervention when they found me in a coma; a near death experience. Tanya said that she and my father knocked on my apartment door in Quincy, Massachusetts at 8:00PM then at approximately 8:45PM and finally at 9:30PM before she called 911 on October 23, 2003. Tanya saved my life when she called the Quincy Fire Department. The fire station was less than a mile away. I will heed her call of need for the rest of my life. I am glad we are friends. You never know who your friends are. It could be your wife and you better make her your best friend because she knows you like a book and you are well read by her. Praise be to the Creator that this women saved my life.

"I am very blessed to be alive and to be a survivor of many near death experiences."

I awoke from the coma two and a half days later. I should have died from the drug overdose for which payment was due immediately. I had foot drop and nerve damage in both feet. When I awoke from my coma, my right foot was twisted from the drugs I had taken in my suicide attempt. I hobbled out of bed, realizing that my suicide attempt was a mistake because I was actually glad to be still alive. The treatment following my near-fatal suicide attempt consisted of rehabilitation for foot drop over the next three months. I was homeless for eight months after my release from the hospital. I should not have ignored my depression by not seeking treatment, which was my responsibility.

My near death experience from my self-induced drug overdose should have killed me and wiped my brain clean like reformatting a hard drive on your computer. My life and brain were spared.

I still had no means of income or family financial support. I spent three months in rehab and the next eight months at a homeless shelter in Cambridge, Massachusetts. That is when I realized that I had not appreciated how much I had before I attempted suicide.

If the Firefighters, EMT's, Doctors and Nurses had not executed their training precisely I may not have made it. I could have died after they found me near death. They all cared about saving my life.

It took this self-induced hurricane; my suicide attempt, when I did not heed the advice given to me to evacuate the coast by properly dealing with personal issues including mental health, eviction, taxes, unemployment, and a failed marriage which lead to three months of rehab for my twisted foot from my drug overdose, then eight months of homelessness. Ironically, these were the first steps to the road of recovery. Years later, I became a person who was kind, polite, giving, no anger, and grateful for all my blessings.

How did I accomplish this? By taking self-help programs and choosing to participate with a positive mental attitude. I had faced death several times and it did not change me until my near-fatal suicide attempt and recovery, I had change before I was able to gain back my self-respect. Self-help programs helped me to become a better person.

It may take you a lifetime to figure which direction you are headed because when you were young you were never given a track to run on. We should take responsibility for the decisions we have made in the past that have brought us to where we are in life. As a young adult can choose to live well if you try to relate to the next message.

You must find a way to live well even if you don't get the proper guidance from your parents because you are the one who is responsible for your own life and the decisions you make. Forget about whom you were; accept who you are, and who you can be. It is your choice.

RESET: CONTROL, ALT, DELETE

I have no doubt there is a Creator and that Creator loves and cares about all of us.

{Gain a pearl of wisdom by clicking on each title. The pearl will be on the top of each page.} I hope that you too will find wisdom in these pearls that have washed ashore as a result of my hurricanes and count yourself a survivor.

"When we change our perception we gain control. The stress becomes a challenge, not a threat. When we commit to action, to actually doing something rather than feeling trapped by events, the stress in our life becomes manageable."

– Greg Anderson

The Cracked Water Pot

– Unknown Author

"A water bearer had two large pots; each hung on the ends of a pole which he carried across his shoulders. One of the pots had a crack in it while the other pot was perfect and always delivered a full portion of water.

At the end of the long walk from the stream to the house, the cracked pot arrived only half full. For a full two years, this went on daily, with the bearer delivering only one and a half pots of water to his house.

Of course, the perfect pot was proud of its accomplishments, perfect for which it was made. But the poor, cracked pot was ashamed of its own imperfection and miserable that it was able to accomplish only half of what it had been made to do.

After two years of what it perceived to be a bitter failure, it spoke to the water bearer one day by the stream. I am ashamed of myself, and I want to apologize to you. I have been able to deliver only half my load because this crack in my side causes water to leak out all the way back to your house. Because of my flaws, you have to do all of this work and you don't get full value from your efforts, the pot said.

The bearer said to the pot, did you notice that there were flowers only on your side of the path but not on the other pot's side? That's because I have always known about your flaw and I planted flower seeds on your side of the path, and every day while we walk back, you've watered them. For two years, I have been able to pick these beautiful flowers to decorate the table. Without you being just the way you are, there would not be this beauty to grace the house."

Save a Life

We could create Life Squads that create awareness, support, and prevention in every Grammar School, Junior High, and High School. The Creator might judge you if you don't try to save the life you could have saved. Why take a chance with your own soul?

Don't allow anyone to have a feeling of hopelessness. There are an infinite number of positive alternatives and possibilities. Be a lifeline for someone who needs your support. We will be undefeated in our pursuit of happiness. Be part of a Life Squad and find someone who needs a friend to lean on.

"We may be judged on what we could have done when you had a moral obligation to help someone in need. You have free will. It is your choice."

– Brian Michael Good

Depression – Homelessness – Shelters

My third pearl washed ashore as a result of my third hurricane. It was self-induced, since I was ignoring my own depression and not accepting a treatment for my mental illness, it was my fault.

When I left the hospital on January 28, 2004, three months after attempting suicide, it was the beginning of my third hurricane. I was homeless for the next eight months in Cambridge, Massachusetts; still challenged and unemployed. I took the subway to a shelter that I had called the day before. I was fortunate to enter a homeless shelter the day I left the hospital but New England was having the coldest winter in a hundred years in the winter of 2004. I arrived at the shelter at 1:30PM with my two suitcases and the caretaker that answered the door told me to come back after 5:00PM because no one was allowed in the Shelter before that time.

I had to carry those heavy suitcases back down those steps while it was snowing. It was one of the coldest days that winter, as the snow covered my suitcases during the next three and a half hours I waited. I was too embarrassed to go anywhere with my heavy suitcases. So, I stood 200 yards away and waited. I really felt homeless that afternoon. I was literally standing in one spot getting very cold because I could not walk very far with my leg braces that I had worn because of my foot drop. Later that day, I entered the homeless shelter where I got out of the cold and snow with a roof over my head. That evening, I was told that it was required to leave the shelter by 8:00 AM every day and not to return until 5:00 PM.

Most days, I walked the streets of Cambridge every day and stopped at the Salvation Army for lunch. It wasn't the best lunch but it was better than no lunch at all and it was a place to get warm. I wore braces for my foot drop every day when I left the homeless shelter, Monday through Friday. On weekends, we were allowed to stay at the shelter during the day with the twenty other people that called the shelter home.

I lived at the homeless shelter for nine months until I got a subsidized apartment through HomeStart, Inc., "a non-profit organization whose mission is to end homelessness in Greater Boston by assisting individuals in obtaining permanent housing and settling into the community, and by developing strategies to address systemic barriers to housing placement.

Many random acts of kindness were given to me during my hospital stay of three months, my nine months of homelessness, and the guidance given to me by the HomeStart, Inc. organization. Without the help of strangers, my recovery would have been quite difficult.

"You will not to be held captive by fear, anxiety or depression."

– Brian Michael Good

Thinking about Death by Suicide

Bad things happen to good people. And sometimes bad things happen for a reason. Someday, in your future, there is going to be a better tomorrow. Know that things will get better. There is an infinite number of possible alternatives and positive outcomes. The answers to your questions are all around you. Sometimes, all it takes is to admit to yourself that you need help to effect a positive change when it comes to your mental, physical or spiritual health. Breathe and stay calm; find a positive solution that will effect change in your life.

Suicide is often referred to as a "permanent solution to a temporary problem". You are not alone and you are not forgotten. Your life will improve. There are those who want to help and support you. I care about you. There are many people who care. How you manage your expectations is the secret to happiness and finding peace in your life. Happiness and peace are for those who seek it. Take control of your life and be a survivor. Talk to someone who cares. Call 800-273-TALK (8255). Studies have proven that with six weeks of proper medical treatment suicidal thoughts will be manageable and subside.

A person who is a little bit insane may be saner than someone who is completely sane. A little bit of insanity gives a person a better perspective on what the difference is between perception and reality. Death by suicide might include any irresponsible, dangerous, or reckless behavior that causes your premature death; except for dangerous situations, someone may encounter in the military, public service, occupation, sports activity, or an unavoidable accident.

If one person cares this much about saving your life then why would even think of killing yourself? Eighty percent of all suicides fail. What, are you crazy? Your free will is taken away. Your life becomes far worse than it is now. Your life is a total mess as a result of your decision. You don't owe me a thing for writing the *Never Surrender Your Soul, RESET: Control, Alt, Delete and Quote Of Wisdom To Live By.*

Only, I ask you from my heart to reconsider killing yourself because I wanted to live when I awoke from my coma of two and one half days. It is a fact that many people that attempt to die by suicide want to live after a suicide attempt. Most people never attempt to die by suicide again because it made their life a living hell.

Stop feeling sorry for yourself because only you can save yourself. Pick yourself up, go take a walk, meet a new friend, or ask someone out on a date. Meet a new friend that will make you laugh.

I made a free will decision to put other people's lives ahead of my possessions. Well worth the sacrifice I made. Nearly everyone wants to live after a suicide attempt. Seek help. Talk with someone. Anybody. It's better than giving up your soul.

Suicide is any self-destructive behavior that results is your death. Life is not only precious but living your life in a developed country is a privileged life compared to living your life in a third world country. There is always someone in the world that would be willing to take your place and fight your fight. They will gladly get on medication that is not readily available in their country, learn to live with your pain, adapt to your depression, and overcome your fears; do not die by suicide and live the rest of your life at peace. This is why death by suicide is an unforgivable act because there are so many others who would love to have your life.

Be honest about your mistakes. Think about the real reasons why you are feeling down. Don't let it bother you if you are up the creek without a paddle. The evil in your life is the abuse you allow others to bestow on you. So, if you are a survivor like me and others like me, just be fearless.

It might be the only way to save yourself from fear. Fear can consume you and spit you out dead. Why die when I wanted to live the moment I awoke from my coma in October of 2003? Why would you kill yourself when there are an infinite number of alternatives and possibilities?

"Free will is our greatest gift after life itself, that being said, Free will must be exercised wisely. As much as is humanly possible."

– Brian Michael Good

Invictus

"Out of the night that covers me,
Black as the Pit from pole to pole,
I thank whatever gods may be
For my unconquerable soul.
In the fell clutch of circumstance
I have not winced nor cried aloud.
Under the bludgeonings of chance
My head is bloody, but unbowed.
Beyond this place of wrath and tears
Looms but the Horror of the shade,
And yet the menace of the years
Finds, and shall find, me unafraid.
It matters not how strait the gate,
How charged with punishments the scroll.
I am the master of my fate:
I am the captain of my soul."

– William Ernest Henley

Play the Hand Life Dealt You

How you play the hand that life has dealt you will define your life and could determine if you meet your destiny.

Do not judge your lot in life and do not over judge yourself. Do not feel sorry for yourself. Stop whining. Do not self-pity. Life can always be worse than it is. Nothing is the end of the world. There is always a way to fix it. Being more positive can help heal life's disappointments. Your perception of what happens in your life and having realistic expectations creates a positive influence in your life. Failures are stepping-stones of success.

"In the middle of difficulty lies opportunity"

– Albert Einstein

I have made many mistakes in my life that were the result of making the wrong decisions and bad choices. I take responsibility for the decisions that I have made in the past that have bought me to where I am in life. We are all human, be comfortable with this fact. Life will always be what you make of it. Forget about whom you were; accept who you are, and who you can be.

Sometimes the hand that life has dealt us is because of the decisions and actions we have made. We realize we dealt the hand ourselves. Only you can change your life.

You will find that the sum of your challenges, hardships, and obstacles will define your human spirit and years later as you reflect on your experiences, you will realize it has become your strength.

"The secret of getting ahead is getting started."

– Mark Twain

"Knowing is not enough; we must apply. Willing is not enough; we must do."

– Johann Wolfgang von Goethe

Never Surrender

I pushed myself so much during the marathon writing of *Never Surrender Your Soul* and *RESET: Control, Alt, Delete* that I should have died many times. I cared that much that you should live. I fed myself to the lions, in a modern sense, becoming homeless for nine months beginning on December 8, 2010 as a result of putting people in need ahead of my needs. My body was totally exhausted but I was always full of energy as I averaged just over two hours of sleep a night from May 2010 to November 2010, going twenty-four to fifty-six hours at a time without sleep. And from November 2010 until April 2011, when I averaged four hours sleep per day. My thoughts kept going, I couldn't stop thinking. It was like going through Boot Camp for you. I should have died for you but the Creator wouldn't let me. Each time approaching death the Creator lifted me.

Was it worth it? Yes, for if I change one life or save just one person from suicide, then I will have paid the Creator for my soul which was a debt due immediately, if I had died from my attempted suicide. I attempted to give up my soul and eternal life. A life for a life. A soul for a soul. I have reclaimed my life and all I had to do was rebuild the fabric of my life. I was destined to attempt to die by suicide, the Creator knew I would write *Never Surrender Your Soul* and *RESET: Control, Alt, Delete*. Well worth the sacrifice I made.

I gave the Creator most of my free will on May 11, 2010 after I went to "Walk to Emmaus," a four-day renewal movement designed for improving relationships with Jesus Christ. I have a non-denominational faith in the Creator. Many people have tried to influence my way of thinking and have taken the fabric of my life from me. The Creator had destined me to live a life of being abused so I would tell you my story.

With my busy schedule I don't always have the time to read the Bible of Faith so I read from *Quotes of Wisdom to Live By*, published by Big Bang Publishing on August 1, 2015; the book I wish I had read before my suicide attempt. I wish I had known about these quotes but then I would not have written *Never Surrender Your Soul*, and *RESET: Control, Alt, Delete*. Go Figure. The Creator works in mysterious ways.

"I am the master of my fate: I am the captain of my soul."

– William Ernest Henley, Invictus

About Brian Michael Good

Brian Michael Good was born in Milton, Massachusetts, the third child of eight. My mother Mary said, I was conceived one month after she had a miscarriage in the first trimester on the night my parents had an argument, which was brought on by the Creator no doubt.

My mother said I had my own language the first year I talked, often doubling my words when I spoke. My first two years in school I went to two different public schools for kindergarten and I was told that I had to repeat kindergarten because my older brother and sister both were kept back in the first grade, which I hadn't even attended yet! The school officials thought it would be better for me socially to repeat kindergarten instead of the first grade. I began my twelve years of parochial education at St. Agatha School in Milton, Massachusetts. There was no such thing as special education so I struggled through grammar school.

At nine years old, I delivered morning and evening newspapers including Sunday delivery. I had one of the largest paper routes in the Boston area. During the summer, I would cut lawns and during the winter, I would shovel snow for extra money. After completing a form and obtaining the required signatures, I received a work permit at the age of thirteen. I started working at a local 7/11 and then at an Italian restaurant when I was fourteen years old.

After grade school, I applied to Boston College High School but my application was rejected. I went to the administration office and asked them what I would have to do to get into the school. The Jesuit from the admissions office told me that if I passed an English and Latin course during the summer then I would be able to start freshman year in the fall. I passed both subjects that summer and was accepted by BC High School. I worked four to five nights a week which paid for my education at BC High. My father made sure I saved fifty percent of the money I made. By the age of twelve, I made my first of two purchases of stock in Admiral electrical appliances.

I graduated from a high school with one of the most rigorous academic programs in New England. I paid for my own tuition and living expenses except for the roof over my head and my mother's home cooked meals by working at an Italian restaurant four to five nights a week. At sixteen and a half, I purchased my parent's station wagon.

I started college when I was twenty years old at University of Massachusetts, Amherst in the spring semester of 1976. I decided to transfer to University of Massachusetts, Boston after two semesters because of the lack of employment opportunities. I tutored eight of my core courses at the University of Massachusetts, Boston where I received a Bachelor of Science degree in Management and Economics having passed my writing proficiency exam on the third attempt which was required before I received my degree. During college, I worked at St. Johnsbury Trucking Company as a spare dockworker, a waiter at a diner, and a bus boy, bar-boy, and waiter at a Holiday Inn. I was living the American dream. There were no obstacles I could not overcome. I paid for my college and living expenses and paid back one hundred percent of my student loans.

In my last semester of college, one course shy of graduating with a double major, I was the head of the U Mass Boston Skydiving club. I was well known, considering I was a student at a commuter campus. Then the doctors at the New England Medical Center, Boston, told me I had a six-pound inoperable tumor between my abdomen and spine that was doubling every two months. The cancer would have been twelve pounds, two months after it was discovered, and twenty-four pounds, four months after my cancer was diagnosed.

I have faced death so many times in my life and been within an inch of death only to have survived, that I believe in Creator and spiritual life after death one hundred percent. During my twenties, I had four parachute malfunctions; twenty times the national average for one hundred and forty-seven skydives. My fourth malfunction was the result of the automatic opening device deploying my reserve parachute prematurely at just over 6,000 feet while performing an attached four-way diamond with three other skydivers off the step of a Cessna 182 airplane at 7,500 feet.

I fell asleep at the wheel more than once while driving on road trips of several hundred miles only to be saved by a truck driver's quick reaction and defensive driving that prevented a car accident. More than once on other occasions my subconscious slammed my brakes or turned my steering wheel out of harm's way with no apparent explanation. This has happened often enough in my life that I no longer believe in luck. I believe I am blessed.

On October 23, 2003, I took enough pills to kill an elephant only to survive by a miracle that was Creator's intervention. I prayed to Creator before I attempted suicide. I knew it was wrong, that Creator could have created me as a rock or a tree. I knew it is a blessing to exist as a human no matter what happened to me, or what kind of life I lived. There are always people in this world with less than we have and with more hardship than we will ever experience and they do not attempt suicide. I asked for forgiveness for what I was about to do. I knew that it was wrong to attempt death by suicide; it was the opposite of the positive mental attitude I had nearly every day of my adult life. Was I brain dead before or after I took those pills? I was predestined to attempt suicide so I would care about suicide. I do believe that it was "divine providence" when I was found thirty minutes before my death by suicide. The Creator knew I would write *Never Surrender Your Soul*, and *RESET: Control, Alt, Delete*.

My estranged wife Tanya told me she came with my father and knocked on my apartment door at eight o'clock, at eight forty-five, and at nine-thirty, thirteen hours after I overdosed on the pills that I was prescribed. I always say the Holy Spirit brought them to my door three times. After three attempts knocking on my door, they called 911. The Quincy Massachusetts Firefighters and EMTs found me in a coma after I overdosed on forty-four pills that should have killed me within several hours. The EMT told Tanya, that when they found me I was thirty minutes from death.

During a three-week period in October 2003, I lost my job and two vans and was told to vacate my apartment with a four-day notice. I spent four days in a county jail for not being able to pay child support for my daughter from a previous marriage. Tanya told me she filed for divorce the day I was released from jail. I was deeply depressed and saw no way out. There was nobody I could turn to for help and I did not know how to reach out to someone. Life no longer seemed worth living when I tried death by suicide.

You must find a way to live even if you suffer from shunning, teasing, gossiping, bullying, shaming, child abuse, sexual abuse, verbal and/or physical abuse. You are the one who is responsible for your own life and the decisions you make.

I now respect the gift that Creator gave all of us, Life. I am very blessed to be alive. There is no doubt that I should be dead.

Today, I will try to stay in the eye of my hurricane where I am safe from the storm around me. I will deal with my hurricanes and struggles in life with no blame or excuses. Nevertheless, my hurricanes keep coming. I gain strength with each pearl of wisdom that washes ashore.

Some of the reasons I attempted suicide included depression, unemployment, eviction, and social pressures. A psychologist once told me that I had plenty of reasons to attempt suicide but not to try it again. That must have meant that I choose to allow a sane man (me) to be driven to an insane moment when I took all those pills.

I started writing a journal in July 2008 because of the continued absence of my daughter in my life and my best friend died in January 2008 while under the influence of alcohol and drugs when his RV hit a utility pole. After the accident he stepped on a live wire and died a few days later. My experiences in life inspired me to write *Never Surrender Your Soul* and *RESET: Control, Alt, Delete* books simultaneously over a period of six-years. You cannot rush inspiration, for inspiration comes from the body, mind, soul, and the cosmos.

I have a non-denominational faith in the Creator. Many people have tried to influence my way of thinking. The Creator had destined me to live a life of being abused and I chose to accept that. Some of my most controversial epiphanies were typed in the relaxing atmosphere that Starbucks offers in Gulf Breeze, Florida.

I would not have completed the first leg of my destiny without the acceptance and patience the south has learned to endure from the northern wind that blows into the Emerald Coast from season to season. I am blessed to live in a country where people believe in giving others a second chance.

The gift of acceptance was from my community listening to my story that was presented with the force of a hurricane. The south has converted my lost soul and thus saved another Yankee.

The true thanks goes not to me but to residents of the Santa Rosa and Escambia Counties for their enduring patience of listening to a long-winded but faithful northern wanderer, for without their guidance I may not have latched onto my dream of the redemption of my soul.

Nutricare Plus,
Tattoo You AfterCare,
and Best To Live

Since 2001, *Nutricare Plus* and now *Tattoo You Aftercare* continue to market natural health and healing by offering special formulated skin care products, herbal remedies and pure emu oil for the body, mind, and spirit using only the highest quality of herbal, natural, and organic ingredients.

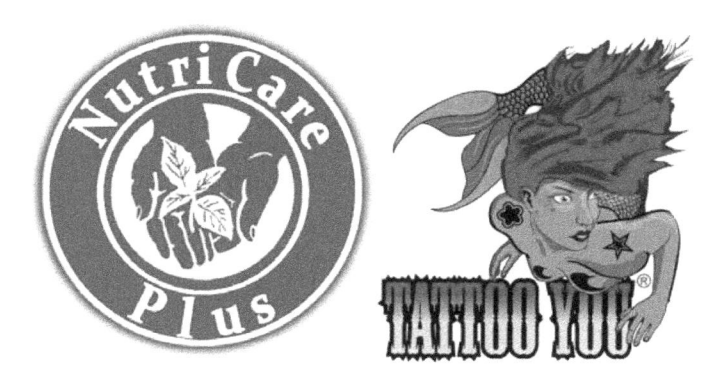

----

www.NutricarePlus.com/Testimonials

Shirley Wood's Testimonial

Esthetician to the Hollywood Stars

Ms. Wood for sixteen years was a staff Esthetician to the Hollywood stars while she was working for Warner Brothers in Burbank, CA consulting with makeup artists and hair stylists. She also was a consultant for prestigious salons in both Beverly Hills and Sherman Oaks, California where she provided esthetic consultation to many famous actors and actresses too numerous to mention.

Shirley Wood has spent her life's journey creating softer, firmer, younger looking faces.

I tried the Nutricare Plus Emu oil followed by their antioxidant serum and antioxidant creams. After two weeks I was convinced that my skin had turned to satin. The derma layer had actually taken on a softer and smoother texture.

I am certainly recommending the Nutricare Plus Pure Emu oil, antioxidant serum and antioxidant creams for skincare to all my clients in both Hollywood and throughout the world.

Now you too can enjoy the soothing and refreshing rejuvenation experience and have "Skin that loves to be touched" by Smooth Fusion ®.

BEST TO LIVE

You are not alone and you are not forgotten.

Best to Live, is a 501(c)(3) non-profit, whose goal is to be an outreach initiative providing answers, information, and provide resources for health needs and overall wellness for anyone who needs to survive emotional, mental, or physical stress.

We hope anyone who has been exposed to violence, abuse, extreme stress, or loss of an important person will seek us out if you need a friend to lean on.

The *Best to Live* logo has the Seed of Life symbol behind the text. The blue hues indicate willingness to see solutions in everything.

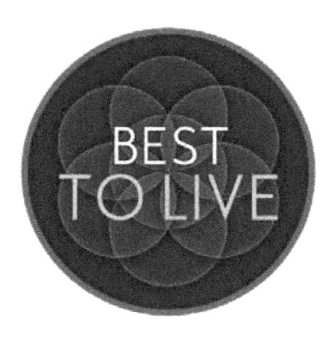

Never Surrender, Be a Survivor,
SURVIVE one day at a time
knowing that it is Best to Live

Take the "*Best to Live LemonAid Challenge*"
to Help Stop Self-Harm

We need to talk about lemons in other words, Help Stop Self-Harm. We would like you to take the "LemonAid Challenge" as a way to raise money for the *Best to Live* Non-Profit. We challenge you to eat three slices of lemon or donate $10.00 to *Best To Live*.

> aid alone anyone best
> besttolive **challenge** cutting
> dollars **donate** donatetenusd
> donatetobesttolive **eat** eighty
> forgotten harm help hopes
> involves **lemon**
> lemonaidchallenge live
> money needs **non-profit** object
> percent provide raise self self-
> harm sharp skin **slices** stabbing
> stop stop-self-harm stress support taking talk
> **wedges**

Donate to Best To Live, Non-Profit, and tweet your support at "#B2LLemonAidCHL"

"When life gives you lemons, make lemonade" is a proverbial phrase used to encourage optimism and a can-do attitude in the face of adversity or misfortune. Lemons suggest bitterness, while lemonade is a sweet drink."

— "When life gives you lemons, make lemonade," from *Wikipedia, the free encyclopedia*

Eighty percent of self-harm involves stabbing or cutting the skin with a sharp object. By taking the "LemonAid Challenge," we can show our support for anyone who self-harms by eating three slices of lemon. This will show that they are not Alone or Forgotten, in the hopes that they will eat a few wedges of lemon before they Self-Harm, hoping they will forget why they were about to cut themselves.

Social Media Links

Brian Michael Good: Author | Writer | Entrepreneur

Meet the Author: www.BrianMichaelGood.com
Twitter: www.twitter.com/1PearlofWisdom
Facebook: www.facebook.com/profile.php?id=100000235296330
LinkedIn: www.linkedin.com/profile/view?id=386147212

Best to Live Foundation, a 501(c)(3) not-for-profit

Website: www.BestToLive.org
Twitter: www.twitter.com/Best2Live
Facebook: www.facebook.com/Best2Live

Spiritual & Personal Growth Self-Help Books

Facebook: https://www.facebook.com/pages/Spiritual-Personal-Growth-Self-Help-Books/357581144409444

Tattoo You AfterCare: Tattoo, Piercing, and Organically Made Skincare Products

Website: www.TatsYou.com/Tattoo-You
Twitter: www.twitter.com/TatUAftercare
Facebook: www.facebook.com/pages/Tattoo-You-AfterCare/307399982774862
Pinterest: www.pinterest.com/TatUAfterCare
Instagram: www.instagram.com/TatUAfterCare
Vine: www.vine.co/u/1205160774373654528

NutriCare Plus: Best Organic and Natural Skincare Products

Website: www.NutriCarePlus.com
Twitter: www.twitter.com/NCPCARES
Facebook: www.facebook.com/NutriCarePlus
Pinterest: www.pinterest.com/NutriCarePlus
Instagram: www.instagram.com/NutriCarePlus
Vine: www.vine.co/u/1202132242860838912

Social Media Connections

The Game of Life Club – TechLevel33Capstone*
www.facebook.com/groups/1415435548766721

Self Help Blogs to Transform your Life
www.facebook.com/groups/SelfHelpBlogsToTransformYourLife

Health, Well-being & Spirituality USA/Canada
www.facebook.com/groups/Health.Wellbeing.Spirituality.USA

Good-Positive-Effective
www.facebook.com/groups/167725706707703

Project happy soul
www.facebook.com/groups/projecthappysoul

Purely Positive
www.facebook.com/groups/384161124949305

Universal Power Healing
www.facebook.com/groups/universalpowerhealing

Expressions of Light and Love
www.facebook.com/groups/www.brianexton

Destination Health, Mind & Soul
www.facebook.com/groups/19303310083623

Friends For All (A Place For Friends & Support)
www.facebook.com/groups/657913414310381

Bipolar/Borderline/Self-Harm/Depression SUPPORT
www.facebook.com/groups/bbsds

Broken Hearts/suicide support/depressed people who need help
www.facebook.com/groups/1476448102586218

Bipolar Awareness and Support
www.facebook.com/groups/1535872206658543

Mental Health Support & Rehab Center
www.facebook.com/groups/713323205410037

Anxiety Chat Group – Private
www.facebook.com/groups/anxietychatgroup

Depression, Suicide Help, Mental Health Support!
www.facebook.com/groups/920528147981916

Depression and Suicidal Help for all
www.facebook.com/groups/300147313515025

Suffering from Panic/Anxiety/Depression
www.facebook.com/groups/340592552791359

I'm not a fighter… I'm a warrior!!!
www.facebook.com/groups/344265405781733

Empath Support Group
www.facebook.com/groups/empathic

Thank You

No person is an island if they want to succeed. I would like to thank the following people who helped me through my journey of writing:

- Helga Holscher who I met in 2008 and who reviewed my journal in early 2009 gave me much needed encouragement.
- Stacie Morgan, even though she was working on her novel in the research stage, reviewed my writings and gave me suggestions that helped me to begin to pull together some initial ideas that proved helpful in the creation of the book's vision in 2010.
- Bryan Hunt, a great talent, who I would like to recognize for his strong work ethic. Bryan has a college degree in Animation. He helped me over several years with my passion for organic and natural skincare by creating the numerous labels, brochures and advertising I needed created. His expertise certainly helped keep my hope alive.
- I would like to thank Nataliya who gave me the title for *RESET: Control, Alt, Delete*. No human is an island if they want to be successful.
- I would like to thank Shelter, Inc. Cambridge, Massachusetts HomeStart, Inc., Cambridge, Massachusetts, and the Waterfront Rescue Mission, Pensacola, Florida for providing a roof over my head when I was a person of need.

- In addition, I would like to thank Laurie Callihan, Dara Rochlin, Christine Rice, and Charlene Truxler, who assisted me in the editing process during various stages of *Never Surrender Your Soul*, *RESET: Control, Alt, Delete*, and *Quotes Of Wisdom To Live By*, and all the people that helped me through my troubled times when I needed to lean on someone the most.

The Boot Camp

    The Boot Camp is for a quick read, containing quotes/passages from *Never Surrender Your Soul* and *RESET: Control, Alt, Delete*. Hopefully you might choose to revisit for further contemplation. If you wish to read more of my quotes I suggest you read my third book Quote Of Wisdom To Live By.

"There's more to well-being than living a spiritual life, it's the state of our planet's future. A spiritual person cares about the environment and sustainability. Being spiritual includes protecting the natural environment by practicing the 7R's…

Reduce your carbon footprint.
Rethink, *Refuse*, *Repurpose*, and *Reuse* items before you discard.
Recycle items that you discard.
Reclaim hazardous waste properly at an eco-collection facility. (Free of charge.)"

– Brian Michael Good

"Changes or events that happen in your life can be fixed or healed with a positive mental attitude. A choice. But when your life is over; it never comes back and you'll never know you could have made it to where you once thought was impossible. Again, a choice."

– Brian Michael Good

"A person who is a little bit insane may be saner than someone who is completely sane. A little bit of insanity gives a person a better perspective on what the difference is between perception and reality."

– Brian Michael Good

"Your children are born with free will. You cannot control their free will without consequences. You are meant to be their guides. If you read your children stories about angels or stories of virtues from a suitable book for children until the age of reasoning, they will learn many important life lessons that will help reinforce good behavior in your children as they mature. Positive reinforcement works far better than any form of discipline that causes excessive fear or anxiety in your child's development."

– Brian Michael Good

"You can do all the right things and still have bad results. Bad things happen to good people and sometimes bad things happen for a reason. Someday, in your future, there is going to be a better tomorrow. Know that things will get better. How you manage your expectations is the secret to happiness and finding peace in your life. Happiness and peace are for those who seek it. Take control of your life and be a survivor. Forget about who you were; accept who you are, and who you can be."

– Brian Michael Good

"Any product labeled American Made should include a customer service center that is answered by Americans in the USA. American Made and Serviced. Now that would create some real jobs numbers."

– Brian Michael Good

"The truth about gossip is the misinformation that is created can influence a teenager or anyone else' decision to die by suicide. Gossip can kill someone emotionally, mentally, physically and spiritually.

If you participate in the gossip you will be part of the chain of gossip that caused another person to repeat it after you. You may not know that the gossip that you participated in is spreading like fire. You may never know how far your gossip has traveled. If the gossip doesn't start in the first place or if you decide not to participate by refusing to listen to gossip; then the wildfire won't grow rapidly and the firefighters called the peacemakers don't need to be called into action to put out the flames.

You may not believe you will pay for your gossip. You might not even know that you need to repent. Everyone that participates in the gossip is at fault. If you gossip about someone then God may judge you. God considers the weak to be his special children even if they are adults. If you gossip repeatedly, you do not have God in your heart and you just don't get it! You may be surrendering your soul."

– Brian Michael Good

"How can an awakening do you harm unless you have not awoken."

– Brian Michael Good

"How you play the hand that life has dealt you will define your human spirit. Do not judge your lot in life and do not over judge yourself. Do not feel sorry for yourself. Stop whining and have no self-pity. Nothing is the end of the world. Life can always be worse than it is. There is always a way to fix it. Being more positive can help heal life's disappointments. Your perception of what happens in your life and having realistic expectations creates a positive influence in your life."

– Brian Michael Good

"Mind over matter. If it matters, you will put your mind to it. The mind is capable of solving anything that matters."

– Brian Michael Good

"Life's journey often requires great courage to overcome our greatest fears."

– Brian Michael Good

"If you do not try to change your world, your world will change you."

– Brian Michael Good

"Fear not. Never look back, never give up, never stop trying, never quit, not even a bit."

– Brian Michael Good

"It is part of our human nature to question what we know and what we don't know."

– Brian Michael Good

"Tomorrow is full of promise if you prepare for today."

– Brian Michael Good

"Everyone needs a chance to be fulfilled with acceptance, which is the impetus to heal old wounds."

– Brian Michael Good

"A positive attitude influences our behavior and dictates a successful approach."

– Brian Michael Good

"Rather than listening to the person with anger in their voice, empower yourself by listening to your inner voice of reason."

– Brian Michael Good

"A book is food for thought… By reading a well written book you will reap pearls of wisdom and have a lifetime of meals."

– Brian Michael Good

"A spiritual or personal growth book can help you change your perspective allowing you to infuse new activities into your life. Life's most valuable pearls of wisdom that are nourishment for the body, mind and soul are often found in books."

– Brian Michael Good

"Humans have become more logical, facts build our knowledge and belief system. A logical person gathers facts and does not rely on faith alone."

– Brian Michael Good

"No one should resolutely affect your pursuit of the truth."

– Brian Michael Good

"A person should weigh all twelve of the universal values to live by equally, following one value and not another is as if you follow none of them. The true lesson gained from having good values comes from valuing the rights of others, not just your own."

– Brian Michael Good

"Life's experiences are not woven with a constant thread; Life in our world is constantly changing. We must repurpose what we have endured and the lessons we have learned; creating a renewed sense of hope. Life is what it is. The question is: what are you willing to do to change your life?"

– Brian Michael Good

"No human is an island if they want to be successful."

– Brian Michael Good

"We are gravitating towards building a belief system that is constructed mainly on materials based on facts."

– Brian Michael Good

"I believe that the best defense against – giving up your Soul – "your very essence" – is your choice of a belief system based on faith, hope, knowledge, reason, and logic."

– Brian Michael Good

"Death by suicide might include any irresponsible, dangerous, or reckless behavior that causes your premature death; except for dangerous situations, someone may encounter in the military, public service, occupation, sports activity, or an unavoidable accident."

– Brian Michael Good

"Respect, like your reflection, must be projected first (good manners) in order to see the same reflection of respect returned."

– Brian Michael Good

"Children are not always mature enough to follow advice but often learn from the example of others."

– Brian Michael Good

"You must find a way to live well even if you don't get the proper guidance from your parents because you are the one who is responsible for your own life and the decisions you make."

– Brian Michael Good

"Each individual should focus on their own personal spiritual life, aware that they may be surrendering their soul in the judgment or treatment of others."

– Brian Michael Good

"Are we that gullible or should we call the story of how Adam and Eve were created as told in "The Book of Genesis" mind control?"

– Brian Michael Good

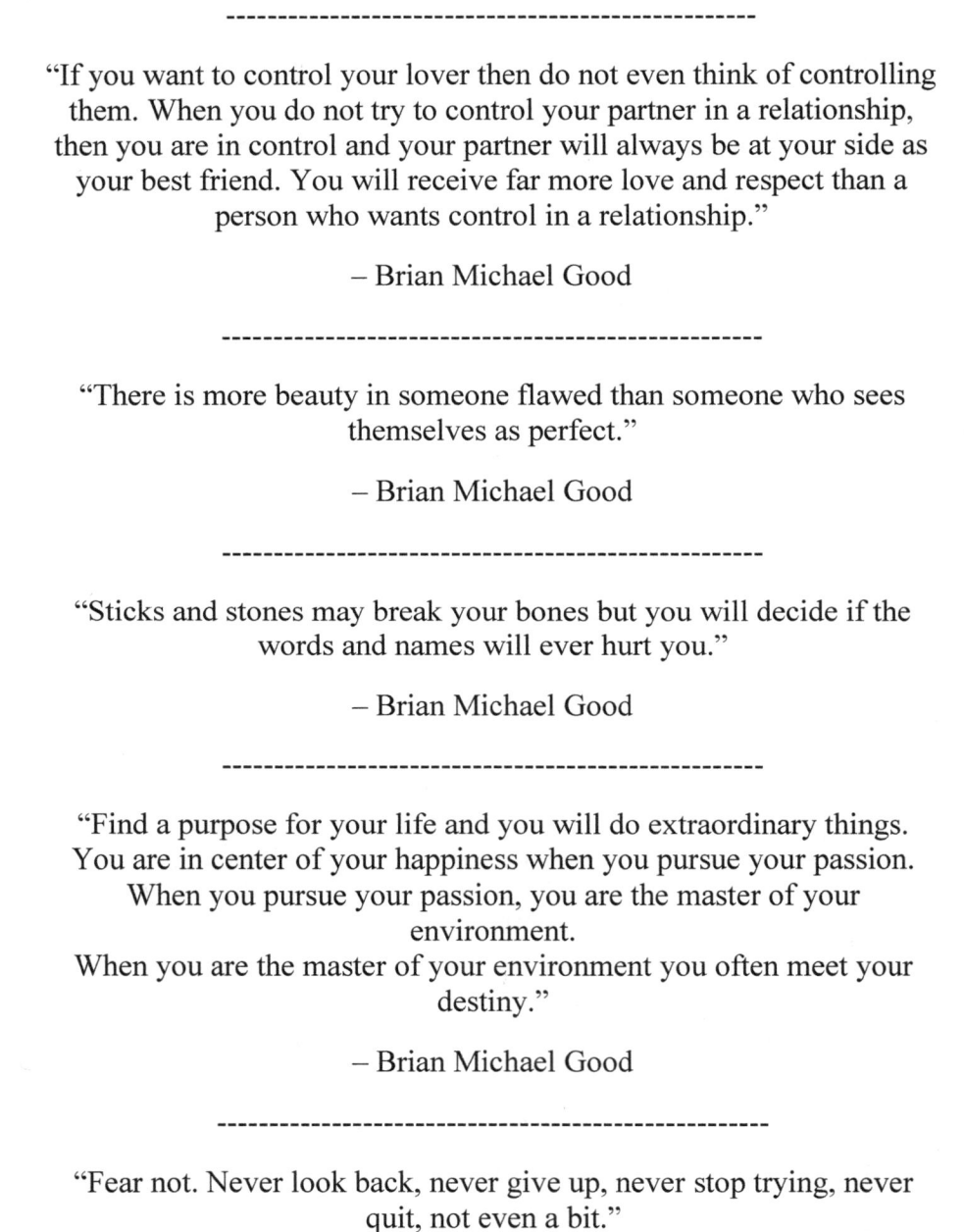

"If you want to control your lover then do not even think of controlling them. When you do not try to control your partner in a relationship, then you are in control and your partner will always be at your side as your best friend. You will receive far more love and respect than a person who wants control in a relationship."

– Brian Michael Good

"There is more beauty in someone flawed than someone who sees themselves as perfect."

– Brian Michael Good

"Sticks and stones may break your bones but you will decide if the words and names will ever hurt you."

– Brian Michael Good

"Find a purpose for your life and you will do extraordinary things. You are in center of your happiness when you pursue your passion. When you pursue your passion, you are the master of your environment.
When you are the master of your environment you often meet your destiny."

– Brian Michael Good

"Fear not. Never look back, never give up, never stop trying, never quit, not even a bit."

– Brian Michael Good

"Fear is a choice. Feeling paralyzed with fear is not an option. Just be fearless. It might be the only way to save yourself from fear. Fear can consume you and spit you out dead."

– Brian Michael Good

"Sometimes failure or defeat is not an option. You can allow your experiences to destroy you or redefine you. No one can defeat you. You can only defeat yourself."

– Brian Michael Good

"Today, I will try to stay in the eye of my hurricane where I am safe from the storm around me. I will deal with my hurricanes and struggles in life with no blame or excuses. But my hurricanes keep coming. I gain strength with each pearl of wisdom that washes ashore."

– Brian Michael Good

"Take responsibility for the decisions that you have made in the past that have bought you to where you are in life."

– Brian Michael Good

"Why would you kill yourself when there are an infinite number of possible alternatives and positive outcomes?"

– Brian Michael Good

"What you choose today, you live with tomorrow."

– Brian Michael Good

"I have come to realize that without the engine; the body, getting a tune-up; the driver, the mind, cannot get where it wants to go in life very well. A healthy mind begins with a healthy body and vice versa."

– Brian Michael Good

"Challenges, hardships and obstacles are what life is all about and if you face them with a positive attitude; you will find that it takes half the effort to overcome them. You will find that the sum of your challenges, hardships, and obstacles will define your human spirit and years later as you reflect on your experiences you will realize they have become your strength."

– Brian Michael Good

"Meeting your destiny doesn't happen without a plan, a plan doesn't happen without a purpose, a purpose doesn't happen without finding your passion, a passion isn't discovered without the pursuit of activities that you enjoy."

– Brian Michael Good

"We are all human, be comfortable with this fact."

– Brian Michael Good

"Tomorrow becomes Today when Today becomes Tomorrow."

– Brian Michael Good

"You will not to be held captive by fear, anxiety, or depression."

– Brian Michael Good

"Sorry means nothing if a person takes no future action to avoid being sorry again."

– Brian Michael Good

"It is nice to be popular but it is popular to be nice."

– Brian Michael Good

"There is no such thing as luck; everything good we experience in our lives is a gift and a blessing."

– Brian Michael Good

"Never let your attitude be the reason for your failure."

– Brian Michael Good

"Find me and you will find yourself."

– Brian Michael Good

"I love you with all the love I have gathered in my lifetime."

– Brian Michael Good

"No one is all good nor is one person all bad."

– Brian Michael Good

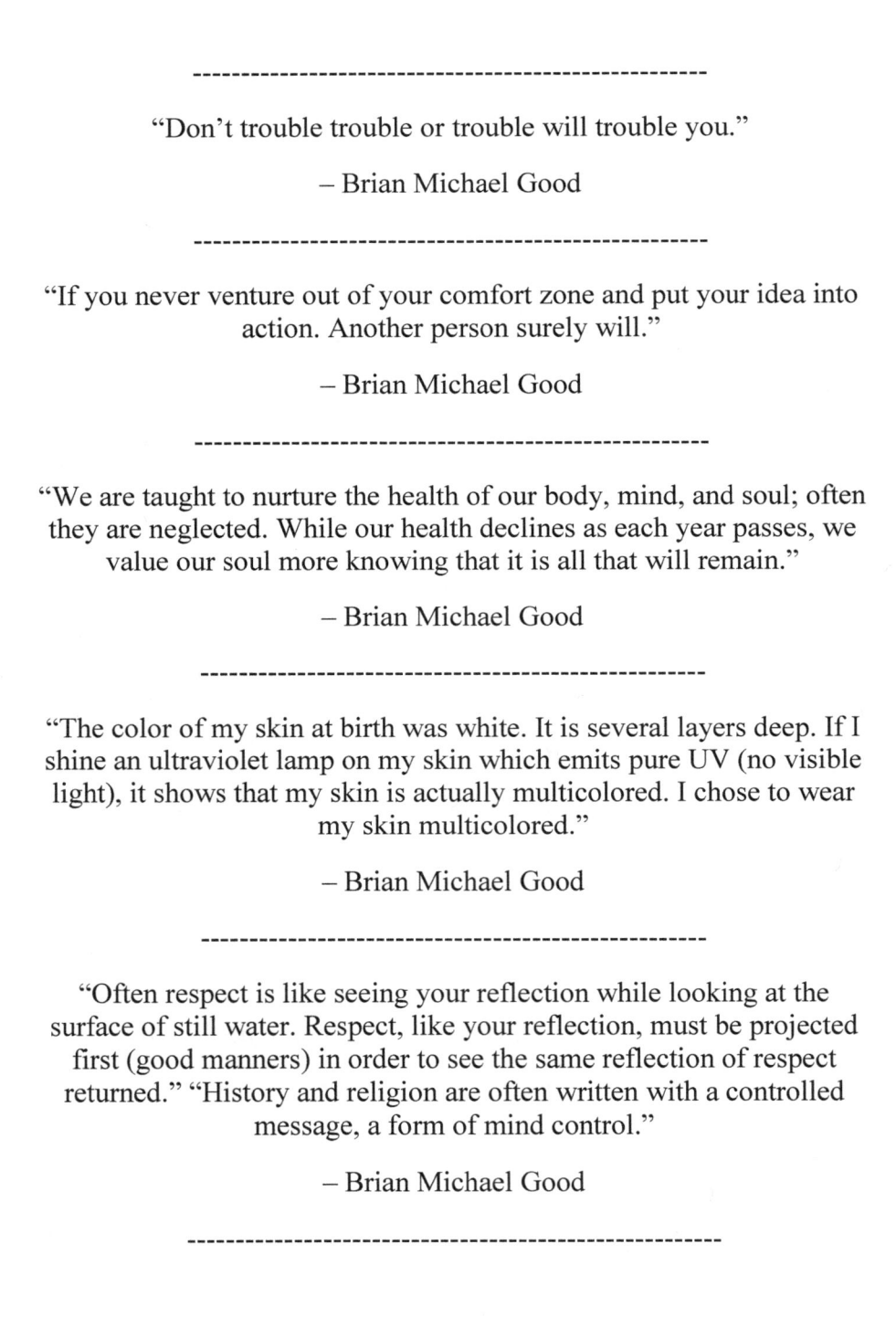

"Don't trouble trouble or trouble will trouble you."

– Brian Michael Good

"If you never venture out of your comfort zone and put your idea into action. Another person surely will."

– Brian Michael Good

"We are taught to nurture the health of our body, mind, and soul; often they are neglected. While our health declines as each year passes, we value our soul more knowing that it is all that will remain."

– Brian Michael Good

"The color of my skin at birth was white. It is several layers deep. If I shine an ultraviolet lamp on my skin which emits pure UV (no visible light), it shows that my skin is actually multicolored. I chose to wear my skin multicolored."

– Brian Michael Good

"Often respect is like seeing your reflection while looking at the surface of still water. Respect, like your reflection, must be projected first (good manners) in order to see the same reflection of respect returned." "History and religion are often written with a controlled message, a form of mind control."

– Brian Michael Good

"At some point in your life, you may wonder if your soul is hanging by a thread. This thread is the conduit in which your belief system flows defining your human spirit and binding to the fabric of your soul. Religious, Philosophical, and Ideological fibers are spun into a single strand giving strength to your beliefs. It is this thread's strength that allows you to be broad-minded and even-handed. Be aware that you may be surrendering your soul in your judgment or treatment of others."

– Brian Michael Good

"You cannot rush inspiration, for inspiration comes from the body, mind, soul, and the cosmos."

– Brian Michael Good

"When you meet another person or when two or more are gathered you will have the opportunity to create the gift of acceptance, the epitome of what humanity should be! The higher you raise yourself in the better treatment of others, the better view you will have of the future."

– Brian Michael Good

"Eternal life has just as much to do with what we do right as what we do wrong."

– Brian Michael Good

"We are powerless when the wind, water, waves, and ice are the agents of the erosion of our beaches that bring changes to our shorelines. We have the power to do something when we allow fear, anxiety or depression to be the agents of the erosion of our hope that affects our emotional, mental, physical or spiritual health. A choice."

– Brian Michael Good

Book Offer

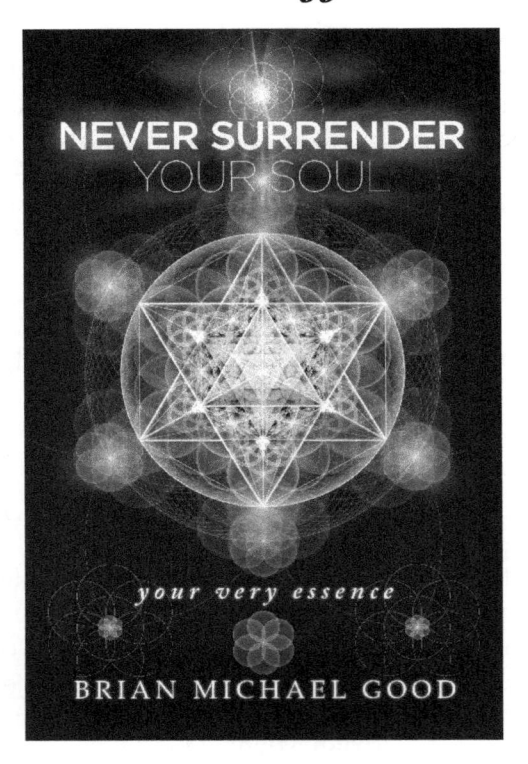

Never Surrender Your Soul – your very essence

Here is the link to visit the book page*:*

www.authl.it/B00RKW5U2O?d

If you wish for personal – spiritual growth and fulfillment in your life and less fear, it is possible! Never Surrender Your Soul unlike other self-help books is written specifically to help you to find the encouragement, strength, and spiritual growth that you will need to change your perspective with less mind control so you can live a hopeful life that creates a path with less fear.

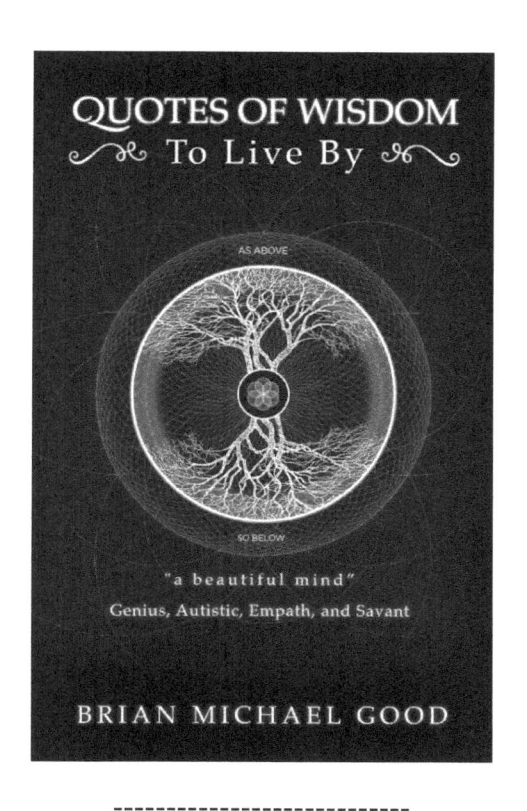

Quotes of Wisdom to Live By

Here is the link to visit the book page:

www.authl.it/B00ZYX4FW2?d

Time is in short supply. Recharge your life with over 365 quotes. Learn how to rise from the ashes of defeat. Life's most valuable pearls of wisdom that are nourishment for the body, mind and soul are often found in books.

"Quotes Of Wisdom To Live By" contains pearls of wisdom for daily living to encourage and guide you through the difficult and challenging days in your life.

"Quotes Of Wisdom To Live By" presents quotes of wisdom thematically arranged. It provides the reader encouragement, comfort and peace by finding the right words of wisdom at the right time.

Join our email list

www.BrianMichaelGood.com/contact-me

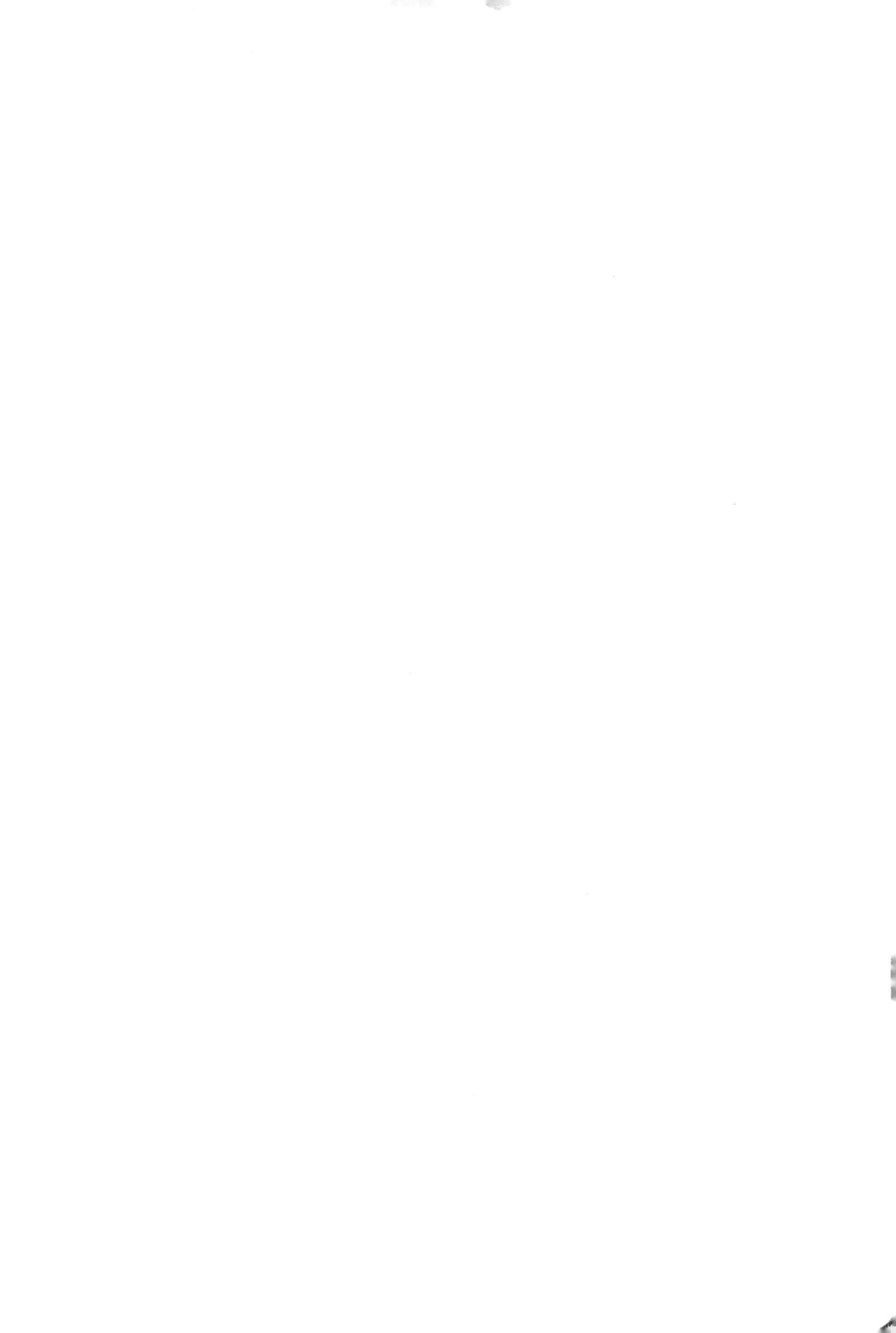

Lightning Source UK Ltd.
Milton Keynes UK
UKHW04f1831220718
326107UK00001B/62/P

9 780986 252761